EXERCISING
IN
BED

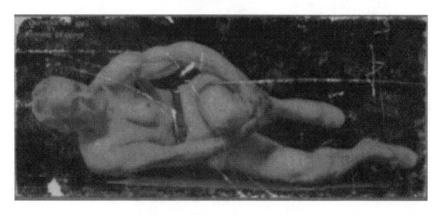

SANFORD BENNETT

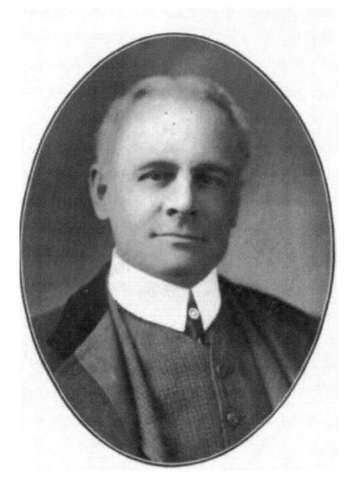

Sanford Bennett

All muscles and all organs increase in size, strength and elasticity when properly exercises. This is the secret of health, strength, elasticity of body, and longevity of life.

Exercising in Bed

The Simplest and most effective
system of exercise
ever devised

By SANFORD BENNETT

DISCLAIMER

The exercises and advice contained within this book is for educational and entertainment purposes only. The exercises described may be too strenuous or dangerous for some people, and the reader should consult with a physician before engaging in any of them. The author and publisher of this book are not responsible in any manner whatsoever for any injury, which may occur through the use or misuse of the information presented here.

Contents

Illustration

Preface

The movements, or muscular contractions and alternate relaxations, described in this system of physical Culture are not specially new, but my adaptation of those exercises, that they may be effectively and systematically practiced under the most comfortable conditions possible (that is, while lying in bed) is to the best of my knowledge, a novel idea and a step in advance in the most important of all sciences, the science of health, strength, elasticity of body, and longevity.

The ease with which the exercises can be performed under these conditions, the small expense of the four simple aids or devices which I use, and the robust health, vital energy, and muscular development which I have obtained at an age when such conditions are very unusual, will commend themselves and invite, at least, a trial. But that trial must be something more than a spasmodic effort made once or twice a week.

To effect any material improvement, determine upon an hour in the early morning when you will commence practice, the number of minutes you will devote to it, and then "stick to it," daily, systematically, regularly, until it becomes a habit; then you will go through the exercises without any conscious effort of the mind, as habit rules our lives, and such a habit will surely bring to your health, strength, and elasticity of body; will increase your vitality an prolong your life.

Sanford Bennett

DEDICATION

To my friend, and companion on many a shooting trip - the happiest days of my long life! Together he and I have climbed the steep quail hills, or waited listening in some rocky canyon to the deep vibrant bay of PEAK mingling with the long drawn bugle-like cry of SCOUT, as, through tangled chaparral, they "cold trailed" some wandering coyote or sneaking cat. And the sharp high staccato notes of NELLIE would break in, when the duct became a trio. The tempo of the wild symphony would quicken, and we would scramble up the rocky ridge to our stand on the high divide.

Together he and I have "lain out" in our blankets watching the glint of the stars in the cloudless California sky; while, far up on the mountain side, the thin weird wail of a prowling coyote alone broke the silence. Then, as the crest of Grizzly Peak reddened in the rising sun, the reedy querulous challenge of the cock quail sounded defiance from sheltering thickets, far and near. The wind, sighing through the redwoods – the pungent smoke of the camp fire – the pure clear air of the early morning; - the joy of it all when one is pulsating with health and lives close of nature.

The picture changes: a bevy of quail is scattered over the brown dry hill side. SHOT and DAN cautiously beat the short sage brush cover. They stop, and stand like statues. I see the quiver of their tense muscles – the gleam of DAN's bright brown eyes. Then, a sharp whir, and the fastest game bird in the world darts like a flash down the gulch. The hammerless goes to my shoulder – the fleecy feathers drift upon the still air. The picture never fades, and years but add to my love of that life.

Al Fischer, crack shot, and companion on many a shooting trip on which we never found the country too rough, the hills too high, or the day too long, I dedicate this book to you, and may the years rest as lightly on your shoulders at sixty seven as they do on mine.

SANFORD BENNETT
Alameda, California, May 1st, 1907.

Clinical Report

By Dr. Carl Renz
966 Sutter Street, San Francisco

Mr. Sanford Bennett, the author of this book, has been the subject of frequent professional examinations during the past eleven years, or, as shown by my office records, first examination made by me February 5, 1895.

When commencing these periodical examinations, he requested that I should keep a careful record of any changes in his physical condition which I might detect, explaining that he had devised a system of muscular contractions and alternate relaxations, which he practiced as he lay in bed, and which he believed would eliminate the worn-out or dead and clogging cellular tissue, hoping that in this way he could rejuvenate his body, which at that period exhibited the conditions usual after the fiftieth year has been passed. His general appearance was that of a man whose vocation had necessitated an indoor life. The outlines of his first record are:

> Height, 5 feet 6 inches.
> Weight, 136 pounds.
> Abdomen, with decided ebonpoint.
> Skin, sallow.
> Varicose Vein on inside of right leg (uses an
> elastic stocking).
> Neck, 14 inches.

Skin, around throat, hanging loose.

Legs, well developed.

Arm Muscles, atrophied and flabby from lack of exercise.

Forehead, deeply lined.

Hair, thin, dark, streaked with gray on crown; quite bald.

Chest Expansion, 3 inches; symptoms of
      Arteriosclerosis slightly developed.

Clinical Examination April, 1906
Or after a lapse of eleven years from first examination

At this date I find a great change in the condition of the muscles, organs, skin, hair, and general health of the subject, who really seems to be rejuvenated.

The hair, now gray, has become quite luxuriant. No indications of former baldness.

The neck, increased to 15 inches, smooth and very muscular; in appearance, the neck of a young man.

Throat, full.

Skin at this point no longer loose and hanging, but firm.

Chin and cheeks, round.

Face, smooth; color, excellent. Appearance of the face is that of a healthy, well preserved man of forty or less. The lines which formerly existed have disappeared.

The development of the arms, chest, back, shoulders, and

abdominal muscles creditable for an athlete of thirty.

Heart, sound; no palpitation or irregularity of pulse.

Chest expansion 5¼ inches.

Waist, 28 inches, No fat around the abdomen; digestion good.

There is a remarkable preservation of tissue integrity and functional activity; the subject has now entered his 66th year, and has all of the elasticity and appearance of a young man.

Under these favorable physical conditions it would be pure speculation to hazard and opinion as to the probable future span of life. The record of my examinations shows a steady improvement of the subject at an age when such improvement is very unusual; this condition seeming to be due solely to the systematic method of muscular contractions and alternate relaxations which he daily practices.

The success, which Mr. Bennett has obtained would seem to be a practical verification of the truth of his theory, "that the secret of health, longevity, and elasticity of the body lies solely in the elimination of dead and worn out cellular tissue, which if allowed to remain in the system would impede the functions and shorten life; and that the only method by which this dead cellular matter can be eliminate is by muscular activity."

Exercising in Bed

I

The Whys and Wherefores

In all ages mankind has endeavored to restore to the aged human body the freshness and elasticity of youth. In olden times these efforts were largely made in the direction of incantations, charms, spells, and even sacrifices of human beings.

Millions of victims have undoubtedly been murdered in the vain hope of obtaining from those victims the life principle, believing that it could be transferred to rejuvenate some aged body.

In the course of my investigations and readings upon this subject, during the past sixteen years, I stumbled across an old work giving an account of the various methods practiced in this direction. Some of these remedies were very laughable; - as pills made from the stomach of a toad killed at some particular phrase of the moon were esteemed of great value, as an aid to longevity. But human sacrifices seem to have been always a favorite method. They were very credulous people in those olden days. Now we are wiser and of courses less credulous. We pin our faith to patent medicines, believing in their virtues, and in the miraculous cures and wonderful properties loudly heralded by their advertisements, just as the people of former days believed in the abracadabra incantations of their magician, pills from a toad's stomach, etc.

It is all very illogical: as, if it were possible to purchase health, strength, elasticity, longevity, and the freshness of youth then the financially richest man would be most generously endowed with these, the real, the greatest natural riches in the world (by reason, of course, of his purchasing power); and the position of drug clerks who had these remedies for sale, would go to a premium, as they would have at their elbow cures for all the evils that flesh is heir to, and, presumably, at cost prices.

If any one of the thousands of hair restorers advertised would perform what is claimed for it in the advertisements, the baldest and richest millionaires in the United States would have a head of hair that would make the spirit of Absalom turn green with envy.

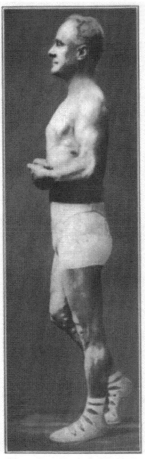

Side View Showing General Development

We are a credulous people: credulous as they were in the days of the magicians who practiced the black art, sacrificing human being in the vain hope of rejuvenating the aged human body, and believing implicitly in the virtues of pills made from a toad's stomach.

We laugh at Ponce de Leon's expedition to Florida, where he hoped to find the fountain of youth in that land of perennial vegetation. We laugh at his foolish expedition, and then go to the nearest drug store and buy Professor Whangdoodle's or some other humbug's elixir, goat lymph, or some decoction of equal value to the delectable pills aforementioned. It is nonsense. You can't rejuvenate the old human body by any medicine, elixir, food, or liquid that you may buy.

The question at once arises; Is it, then, possible to rejuvenate, to any considerable extent, the human body after it has passed, say, the half century limit. Unhesitatingly, and form my own experience. I answer "Yes": and I do not ask acceptance of my statements as to that possibility without proof.

I therefore submit the series of photographs which illustrate this book, showing my present physical condition at the age of 67. I commenced my studies and experiments in this process of rejuvenation when I was entering my 50th year; at that age, I was physically an old man and looked my age, as will be shown by the old photograph, facing page 26.

I am now a younger man physically, and in appearance, than I was when that picture was taken. I find, in speaking of this matter to various interested parties, that they usually refuse to believe that I am as old as I claim to be. There is little difficulty in establishing the fact that I was born in Philadelphia, January 4th, 1841, and therefore have entered my 67th year. The next objection is, that I am abnormally endowed with the vital principle. This is a mistake. My father died of consumption at the age of forty-two, and I inherited that tendency. My family, upon both my father's and mother's side, were not long lived, and my physical start in life was as a nervous, anaemic, frail shred of a child, whom no one ex-expected over the reach maturity. That frail child grew into a slender, nervous, dyspeptic man, and chose the very worst profession in the world for such a physical condition. I became an office man, and the sedentary life of that profession exaggerated a tendency to dyspepsia and its attendant maladies. I became partially bald, was rheumatic, and continually afflicted with minor ailments. It was this unfortunate condition, which impelled me to commence systematically the studies and experiments which have resulted so fortunately for me.

The photographs which faces the 20th page of this book was taken June 4th, 1889, a companion to the one taken February 15th, 1906, appearing on the 22nd page, showing accurately the marked improvement in the face and hair. The rest of the photographs were taken during February, 1906, and the spring of 1907. They are truthful illustrations of my present physical condition. It is unfortunate that I did not preserve any photographs of my physical condition when I commenced to practice the system of exercises described in this book; but I never expected to succeed as I have done. The only photograph taken in the earlier years of my experiments faces page 116. After practicing the exercises nearly five years the years the muscular development shown in this illustration is not very pronounced, but is a great improvement over the physical condition I was in when I commenced.

These pictures are not exhibited as showing any unusual muscular development, nor are they intended for comparison with the physical condition of any youthful athlete, but are presented as specimens of what may be accomplished in the development of an aged

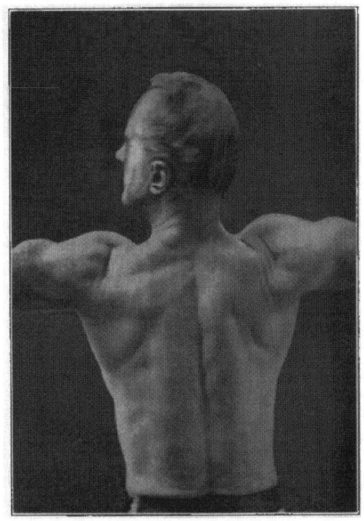

Development of the Shoulders and Arms

body, which, in my case, has been rejuvenated to a very large extent, and this at the age of 67, or 7 years beyond the chloroform limit suggested by Dr. Osler. Regarding that gentleman's statements, I would say that it is my opinion they were based on his own physical condition; and if that is the case I, of course, most heartily agree with him, at least as far as he is concerned, not wishing to disagree with such an eminent scientist. The answer to his statement is that physical age does not depend so much upon the number of years you have spent upon this earth as it does upon how you have taken care of your machinery. Through lack of knowledge, lack of exercise, and violations of the laws of health, it is possible to be physically an old, worn-out man at forty, and a subject for chloroform as the learned Doctor hints at sixty; but, upon the other hand, if the body is kept clear of clogging, worn-out matter, by the simple system described in this look, the walls of the arterial and venous system may remain elastic, and the body at 67 present the appearance of the average athlete of half that age. This much I have demonstrated: What the limit of that condition is I do not know; but at present the most searching investigation of an experienced surgeon does not disclose any sign of physical deterioration. I refer to the report of Dr. Carl Renz, in the first pages of this book.

In my college days I was acquainted with an old trainer of athletes who used to say to us, "Gentlemen, a man is as old as his arteries". I think that was the extent of his knowledge of the physiology or the anatomy of the human body, as he told me in confidence one day that "biled cabbage was bad for men in training', as it got mixed up with their heart and their other works". From my own experience I agree with him as to the effects of biled cabbage on my "other works"; and he had, undoubtedly, condensed a great deal of wisdom in his statement, "a man is really as old as his arteries", for upon the arterial system, from the largest artery to the smallest capillary, a man's physical condition depends. It is evident that the arterial system, or in other words, the plumbing and piping of the human body, must be kept free from all clogging matter. For if this is not done, the muscles and organs are not properly supplied with blood and material for repairs, and will consequently deteriorate and show indications of what we know as age. Such a body could not be healthy or elastic; it would

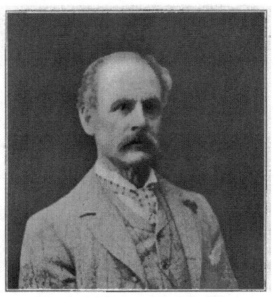

Sanford Bennett at the Age of 50

practically be an old body, and the man or woman in such a condition would be aged, even through his or her years were in number those of youth. On the other hand if the arterial and venous system can be kept clear of such deposits, the walls will remain in the elastic condition characteristic of youth, the heart will pump the blood through those elastic arteries without difficulty, the muscles and organs, being properly nourished, will retain their vigor, and the body preset the appearance of youth at advanced age.

The process of cleansing these arteries, whether the largest artery or the most microscopic capillary, can only be accomplished through the alternate contraction and relaxation of the muscles, that being nature's method of cleansing the body of impurities. It cannot be accomplished by any other means.

To understand how the arterial and venous systems become obstructed with waste or dead matter, it is necessary to have a slight knowledge of physiology, and I will ask you to recall your first lessons in school upon this subject. The human body is composed of billions of cells, or molecules, I prefer the latter term, Webster's definition being "a minute particle"; and these billions of minute particles in aggregate form our bodies. They come into being from the liquid we drink, the air we breathe, and the food we take into the stomach, these materials being converted, by the marvelous process of digestion and assimilation, into cellular, or molecular, life.Each infinitesimal cell has a life of its own, as distinct from the cells or molecules surrounding it as each person is distinct from all others. They come into being, live their brief life, and then die, even as you and I die; and, having become dead matter, should be thrown out of the system. Otherwise they will clog up the arterial, or piping, system of the body. Thus it is easily seen how important it is to free the system of worn-out dead matter; and this cannot be accomplished, and never has been accomplished, by any lymph, serum, elixir, or medicine yet brought before the world. I repeat my assertion that the only process by which it can be done in nature's method, that is, the alternate contraction and relaxation of the muscles; in other words – exercise. In the almost unceasing activity of childhood and early youth we see the manifestation of this plan of removing impurities and dead matter from our bodies.

You can also see the fallacy of the theory of another scientist who created a sensation almost equal to that of Dr. Osler's, by stating, in a widely circulated article, that it was injurious to actively exercise after the age of thirty-five. That gentleman's statement, like Dr. Olser's, was probably based upon a life of mental activity and physical inactivity; result – an old body.

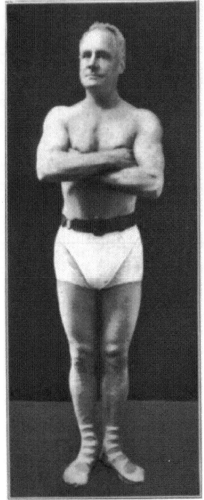

Front View, Showing General Development

Nature's law is this: All muscles, all organs, grow in size, strength, and elasticity when they are properly and persistently exercised; and just as certainly all muscles and all organs of the human body lose these qualities if they are not exercised. It is nature's unalterable law. In short, the secret is exercise; unalterable law. In short, the secret is exercise; exercise, persistent and methodical, from the time you toddle across the floor as an infant, until the shadow falls and the vital cord that connects you with the great reservoir of the life principle snaps, and you step into the mystery beyond.

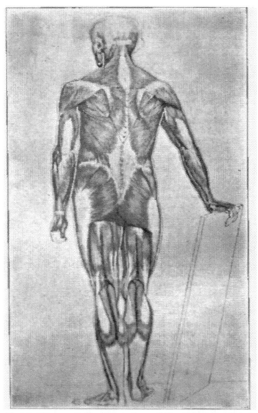

Back View of the Muscles of the Human Body

The most perfect man, possessed of the strongest body the world has ever seen, will surely deteriorate if he does not exercise. This applies to every human being of either sex, of whatever age. There is no exception to the law; and if you would be healthy and prolong your stay upon this earth, you must work for it. There is no other successful method. Dict as you will, stuff yourself with health foods, saturate your system with the most widely advertised preparations for the attainment of health, strength, activity, and longevity, you will not succeed unless you keep the body clear of all dead and clogging matter; and this can only be accomplished though nature's method. There is no substitute.

For the encouragement of those who have reached or passed middle life and think they are too old. I would state that my experience has been that there is not period of life when improvement is impossible. In the cases of several aged people who have sought my advice and adopted my method a beneficial effect has invariably followed. As I have stated, I did not commence to exercise systematically, with the view of the development of the upper part of my body, until I had entered my 50th year; and you will surely succeed if you will follow my instructions and practice increasing your strength, elasticity of body, and length of life upon this earth. You will, most probably, succeed to an even greater extent, and far more rapidly, than I have done, for of the sixteen years that I have passed in experiments, a considerable number have been records of disheartening failures, caused by wrong methods. You will profit by those mistakes and my dearly purchased experience.

Bear this in mind – I emphasize it: all muscles and all organs grow in size, strength, and elasticity if properly exercised; and as surely will they lose those properties, if they are not exercised.

You know the benefit of exercise; but the general impression is that it means joining a gymnasium, or performing a variety of violent motions at unpleasant hours, which, in time, become distasteful and are finally abandoned.

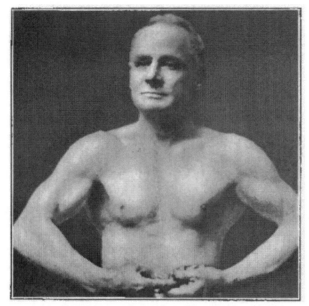

Showing Chest Development

It certainly takes a great amount of courage to get up on a cold morning and go through a series of exercises which may be directed by a physical instructor or a book upon physical training; in fact, more moral courage than I possess. It occurred to me that as this alternate contraction and relaxation of the muscles must be about all that is necessary, the process could be gone though without mechanical appliances, even while lying in bed or in a recumbent position.

To test the theory, I invented a series of exercises of muscular contractions and relaxations, which I practice while I lie in bed in the morning. These movements where so designed as to exercise every part of the body, and I speedily found that equal benefit resulted as though they were practiced in an elaborate gymnasium and in athletic costume.

As the result of my theory and practice the photographs of my present physical condition will give a good idea of the success of my efforts. That success can be yours, if you will practice as I have done.

These rhythmical, muscular contractions and alternate relaxations really constitute a system of muscular pumping which not only eliminates from the parts of body so treated dead cells, worn out tissue, or other clogging matter, but also accelerates the circulation and increases the supply of blood to those parts. And with that additional supply of blood there is an increase of that mystic power, the vital principle. Hence growth, practically a rejuvenation of the muscles.

There is a strong sympathy between all parts of the body one with the other, and any organ, gland, or structure underlying or adjacent to the muscles exercised will be greatly benefited. I have repeatedly demonstrated the truth of this statement in my practice, and can confidently say that improvement is possible at any stage of life, at least up to the age of sixty-seven, for I find that at this period of my life development of the muscles is as readily accomplished by the methods I practice as it was when I first commenced, nearly seventeen years ago.

As all parts of the body can be improved by these exercises, it is evident that a general and systematic method of calling all the muscles into action will result in an absolute rejuvenation of the system; and this is the result I have accomplished in my own person.

The only mechanical appliances that I use are a pair of four-pound dumb-bells, and a board eighteen inches long by four inches broad, to which tow short ropes, eighteen inches in length, are attached, terminating in ordinary pulley-weight handles. This appliance has the effect of a lifting machine in developing the loins and shoulders. It is so used, as I lie comfortably under the bed clothes. In fact, I perform all of these exercises as I lie thus at my ease.

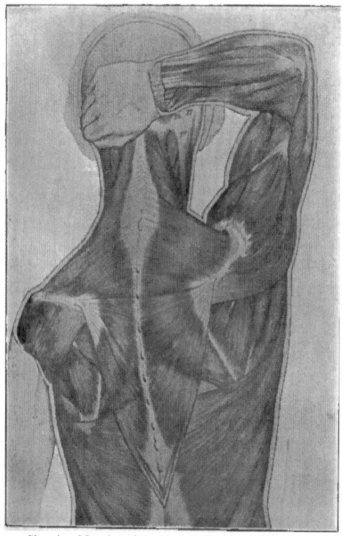

Showing Muscles of the Neck and Arms – Rear View

There are many advantages in this method of exercising. In a recumbent position more muscles can be brought into action than when in an upright position; and I believe that muscles develop, provided the air breathed is pure, more rapidly under these comfortable condition than in the cold, bracing air usually advocated for physical exercise. There is another advantage – the vital force which would be required to prop up your body, if you should exercise in a standing position, can be thrown into any muscles you may be endeavoring to develop (and it is possible to exercise every muscles of the body evenly) without any strain upon the heart. In this recumbent position no danger can result, while it is very possible to overtax this most important of all muscles in the gymnasium.

A regular hour of practice can be set and adhered to. This is very important, as improvement is much more rapid under such conditions than in the irregular manner in which exercise in usually taken; for nature cordially seconds your efforts when they are thus regularly and faithfully put forth.

With these muscles-tensing exercises I have succeed in developing evenly all the muscles of my body, in proof of which I refer you to the photographs exhibited. On the other hand, in the practice of a gymnasium one is very likely to develop one set of muscles and neglect others equally important, as a result of which the body get out of balance, and like any other badly balanced piece of machinery, is not capable of its full efficiency.

It is astonishing the number of exercises that are possible while lying comfortably in bed. Every muscle of the body can be called into action, until a healthy glow results from head to foot from the stimulated circulation, and you realize the full joy of living.

The objection usually raised, is lack of time. Under the usual conditions, possibly; but I take these exercises at a time when I am absolutely idle, and under very comfortable conditions. I wake up at about half-past five, and systematically go through the exercises until, say, half-past six. Then I rise and take a quick, tepid bath. Anyone can perform the exercises. They are simple and effective, and will surely bring to you the greatest riches of the world – health, strength, elasticity, and longevity.

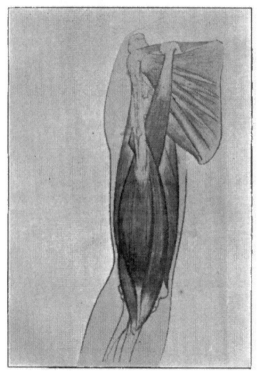

Showing Muscles of the Upper Arm – Side View

Massage Exercise for Developing the Biceps and Triceps Simultaneously with the Loin Muscles
II.

All of these exercises are performed in bed, under cover of the bed clothes

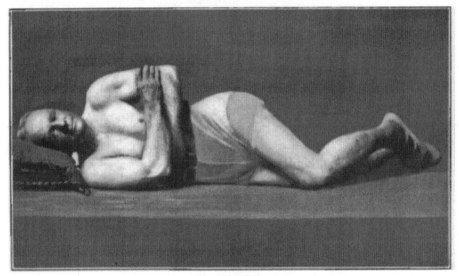

First Position

Massage Exercise for Developing the Biceps and Triceps Simultaneously with the Loin Muscles.

Lying upon your side, extend the upper arm downward, parallel with your body. Grasp it firmly with the opposite hand between the elbow and shoulder; that is, around the biceps and triceps muscles (as in the illustration on this page). Then contract and tense these muscles by bending the arm to the second position (as in the illustration facing page 30). Relax by straightening it to the first position.

While thus alternately contracting and relaxing these muscles of the upper arm, massage them vigorously, both in their tensed and relaxed conditions. The beneficial effect of massage of the muscles while exercising has already been described.

During these movements, exercise the muscles of the loin by throwing the upper hip forward (as in the illustration opposite); then back to the original position. This is an excellent and perfectly safe exercise; it will strengthen and give elasticity to the loin muscles, and its practice will insure speedy development of the upper arms.

The forward movement of the upper hip should be simultaneous with the contraction of the upper arm; commence with five movements, and, as your physical condition improves, increase the number to twenty-five.

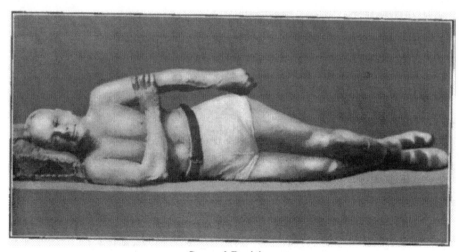

Second Position

Exercise for Developing the Triceps, Or Back Muscles of the Arms
III.

**All of these exercises are perform in bed,
under cover of the bed clothes**

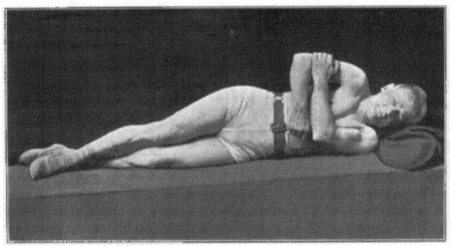

Developing the Back Muscles of the Arms

Exercise for Developing the Triceps,
or Back Muscles of the Arms

Lying upon your side grasp firmly the upper arm, between the elbow and the shoulder, as in the position shown in the illustration facing this page. Pull backwards with the upper arms, at the same time resisting the pull by the firm grasp and downward pull of the lower hand and arm.

Commence with five movements; that is, alternately pulling and relaxing the strain.

I do not know of any gymnasium exercise, aided by mechanical appliances, that will so speedily develop the muscles described. It is a safe, simple, and very effective exercise.

Twisting Exercise for the Development of the Arms
IV.

**All of these exercises are perform in bed,
under cover of the bed clothes**

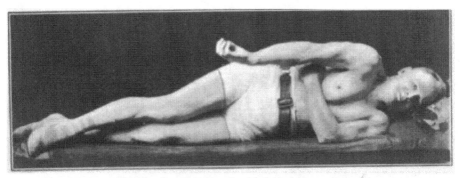

Developing the Arm by Twisting Exercise

Twisting Exercise for the Development of the Arms

This movement brings into action all the muscles of the arms, and is exactly like the exercise of fencing, in which the play of the foils necessitates this twisting motion. The benefits of fencing are well known; but as only the right arm is used by the fencer in his amusement that arm is often unduly developed, while the left is neglected. He is, therefore, in this respect usually ill-balanced.

In lying upon you side, extend your upper arm at full length, parallel with your body, as shown in the illustration facing this page. Clench your fist tightly, that the muscles may be tensed. Twist your arm around toward your body as far as possible without inconvenience; then reverse the movement.

Commence with five or ten movements; that is, twisting the arm backward and forward, as directed.

This is an excellent exercise for ladies who wish add to the symmetry of their arms, as improvement is certain if the practice is persistent. It is, of course, understood that both the right arm and the left must be exercised in this manner; otherwise an unequal development will surely result.

Resistance Exercise for
Developing the Arms
V.

**All of these exercises are perform in bed,
under cover of the bed clothes**

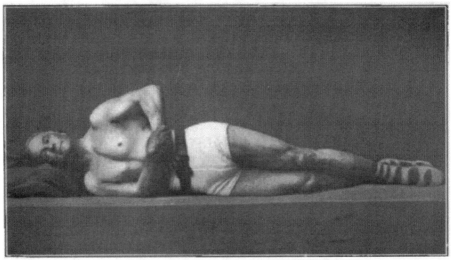

Developing the Arms by Resistance

Resistance Exercise for Developing the Arms

Lying upon your side, as shown in the illustration on the opposite page, grasp the upper wrist with the lower hand and pull upward with the upper arm, resisting that pull with the downward strain of the lower arm. At each movement, that is, in the alternate strain and relaxation of the muscles, turn the wrist slightly, as it lies in the clasp of the hand. In the one position, the front of the wrist should met the palm of the opposing hand; and in the next, the side of the wrist should be presented to it.

This slight change, made by the turn in the wrist, will bring into action another set of muscles, and if you desire to thoroughly exercise the muscular system, do not overlook these apparently trivial changes in position.

To ladies endeavoring to improve the symmetry of their arms, I strongly recommend this exercise. Commence with ten movements, and increase, as your physical condition improves, even to the point of fatigue. Benefit will surely result.

Resistance Exercise for Developing the Fore-Arms VI.

All of these exercises are perform in bed, under cover of the bed clothes

Resistance Exercise for Developing the Fore-Arms

Lying upon your side, grasp the wrist of your lower arm with the upper hand; press with your full strength downward, resisting with upward pressure, as in the illustration on the opposite page.

Commence with five movements; that is, alternately exerting and relaxing the pressure upon the lower wrist; increase, as your physical condition improves, to ten or fifteen. It is a perfectly safe exercise, and will add to the strength of the fore-arm.

This exercise is specially designed for the development of the fore-arm, but you will find that it brings into action and tenses all the muscles of the arm. It should be practiced both upon the right and left side.

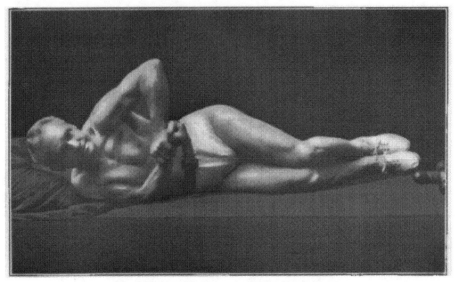

Developing the Fore-Arms by Resistance

Pulling Exercise, for Strengthening the Muscles of the Back and Loins, VII.

All of these exercises are perform in bed, under cover of the bed clothes

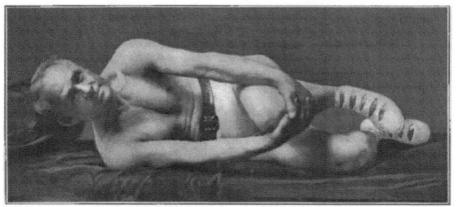

Developing the Back and Loins by Pulling Exercise

Pulling Exercises, for Strengthening the Muscles of the Back and Loins

Lying upon your side, clasp your hands over the upper knee, as shown in the illustration upon this page. Exert your full strength in a steady pull; then relax.

Commence with ten movements (that is, alternately pulling steadily a few seconds upon the bent knee and then relaxing the strain). As you gain strength, increase to twenty-five movements.

The tension will come principally upon the back muscles of the shoulders, but this is also an excellent exercise for the development of the loin muscles, which are brought into action by the effort.

This exercise is perfectly safe, and improvement in the muscles so treated is certain, if the exercise is systematically and regularly practiced.

In all of these exercises, when the position is upon the side, go through the whole series for that side before changing the position. I practice in the order of the descriptions and illustrations.

Single-Arm Pulling Exercise VIII.

All of these exercises are perform in bed, under cover of the bed clothes

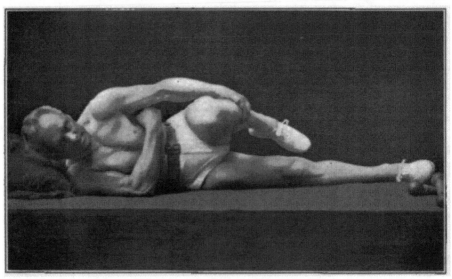

Developing the Back and Loins by single-Arm Pulling Exercise

Single-Arm Pulling Exercise

Lying upon your side, as in the preceding exercise, clasp one hand only around the ankle of the upper leg, as in the illustration upon the previous page. In this position, pull with your full strength, holding the strain for a few seconds; then relax.

Commence with ten movements, (that is, alternately tensing and relaxing by the pulling exercise described), and increase, as your physical condition improves, to twenty-five movements.

You will find the tension of the shoulder muscles in this effort different from the preceding exercise, the strain being across the shoulders as well as downward. This, like the pulling exercise, is perfectly safe; the muscles specially brought into action are those which make up the "neck yoke" and those immediately around and bracing the shoulder sockets. It is designed to strengthen and generally develop the muscles of the back.

Tensing Exercise for the Whole Body
IX.

All of these exercises are perform in bed, under cover of the bed clothes

Tensing Exercise for the Whole Body

There are many deep-seated minor muscles which are not called into activity by the special exercises previously described. The capillaries which should nourish them, and the microscopic veins, by this inactivity, may become clogged, losing their elasticity and efficiency, just as the larger arteries, veins, and muscles will deteriorate under like conditions. It is therefore necessary to bring this dormant machinery into action. To effect this, lie upon your side, fold your arms across your chest, grasp your elbows with the hands, throw your head well back, and stretch your body to its full length, as shown in the illustration upon this page. In this attitude exert at first but half of the strength of your folded arms – the pressure coming upon the elbows, over which your hands are clasped. As you do this, stretch and tense your entire body until it becomes rigid. Hold this position but two or three seconds, as the effect is as though you were lifting a heavy weight. Relax for a few seconds; then repeat the effort. Three or four movements, - that is, alternate tensing and relaxing of the muscles, - as described are sufficient. This exercise will set the blood "tingling in every vein," and, most probably, will be followed at first by perspiration.

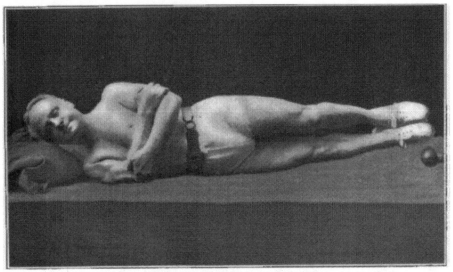

Developing the Whole Body by Tension

Commence the exercise cautiously; exert only half your force in the pressure of the folded arms, and gradually increase, as your strength increases. Commence with not more than three or four movements; increase slowly until you have reached ten, which will be sufficient.

Exercise for Developing the Back and Shoulder Muscles
X.

**All of these exercises are perform in bed,
under cover of the bed clothes**

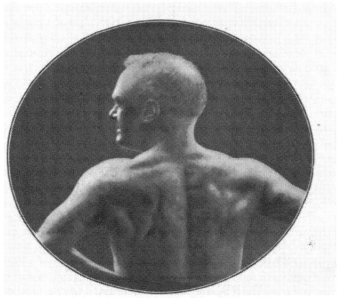

Results of Exercising the Muscles of the Back

Exercise for Developing the Back
And Shoulder Muscles

In this exercise, remain in the same position as that just described, - that is, upon your side with the arms folded across the chest, - bend the head well forward, thus tensing the muscles at the base of the neck, and those surrounding it. Exert your full strain upon the folded arms (the lower part of the body being relaxed); in this position shrug your shoulders up and down. This action will alternately tense and relax the large muscles of the upper part of the neck and shoulders.

Commence with five movements, and increase to, say, fifteen.

This is a very effective exercise, and is without danger of strain. The illustration upon the opposite page illustrates the muscles developed by this method.

Bar Exercise Number I
For the Development of the Muscles of the Arms and Shoulders.
XI.

All of these exercises are perform in bed, under cover of the bed clothes

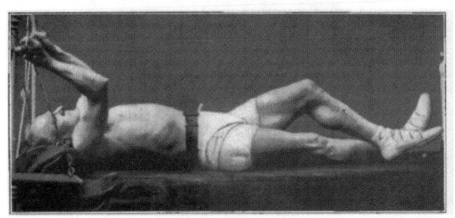

Developing the Arms and Shoulders by Bar Exercise Number 1

Bar Exercise Number I
For the Development of the Muscles of the Arms and Shoulders

Firmly attached across the head-board of my bed is a stout hickory bar 1½ inches in diameter and as long as the head-board is wide.

Lying upon my back, I grasp this bar with both hands, as shown in the illustration upon the previous page. I employ sufficient strength to bring the muscles of my arms to full tension, but not to move the body.

The action is similar to that gymnasium exercise known as chinning the bar, with the difference that I lie upon my back.

Chinning the bar is a favorite gymnasium exercise with young athletes, as its practice usually results in very satisfactory developing the muscles specially called into action; but it places a great strain upon the heart, and becomes therefore a somewhat hazardous exercise as we advance in years.

Commence the exercise with five motions; increase gradually, until your physical condition will warrant twenty-five daily without fatigue or soreness of the muscles.

I weigh, stripped, 140 pounds; the force of the pull would not raise more than half of that weight, therefore the body moves but slightly from its position, while the muscles of the arms and shoulders are thoroughly exercised.

The method I have described is perfectly safe at any age; the pull can be proportioned to your physical condition and the heart will not be overtaxed.

Bar Exercise Number II
Similar to the Foregoing Exercise, with the Exception that but One Hand is Used

XII.

All of these exercises are perform in bed, under cover of the bed clothes

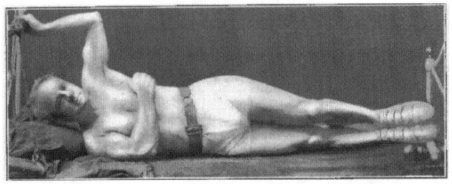

Developing the Arms and Shoulders by Bar Exercise Number 2

Bar Exercise Number II
Similar to the Foregoing Exercise, With the Exception that but one Hand in Used

This exercise is designed to stretch the large muscles immediately surrounding, and below, the arm pit, which do not seem to be so directly called into action when using both arms. The shoulder, in this exercise, is raised higher, and the tension upon the muscles described is more decided. See anatomical plate, facing page 29.

Commence with five movements and gradually increase to twenty five, as your physical condition may warrant.

Exercise for Developing the Muscles of the Sides and Loins
XIII.

**All of these exercises are perform in bed,
under cover of the bed clothes**

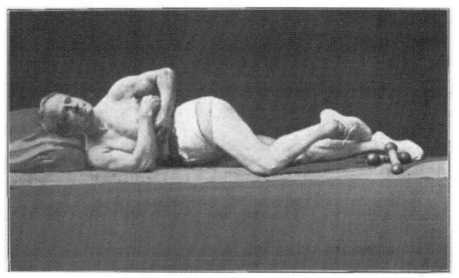

Developing the Sides and Loins

Exercise for Developing the Muscles
of the Sides and Loins

Lying upon your side, as shown in the illustration on this page, raise the head and both feet at once; this will contract the side muscles of the loins and the large muscles which descend from immediately below the arm pits into the loins. The exercise will also strengthen the muscles of the stomach. It is an excellent one, but somewhat fatiguing.

Commence with but three movements. Six or seven will probably prove the limit to which you will care to go, as the strain is equivalent to lifting a heavy weight by the muscles described. Therefore, if adopted, the exercise must be commenced and practiced with caution.

Exercise for Strengthening the Lower Abdominal Muscles
XIV.

**All of these exercises are perform in bed,
under cover of the bed clothes**

Exercise for Strengthening the Lower Abdominal Muscles

In the human being the lower abdominal muscles, which cover that part of the abdomen lying between the hips and lower portion of the pelvic bones, are subject to a continuous strain, as they support the heavy viscera within. If they become weakened through inaction they will relax, and that unsightly condition known as "pot bellied" may result. A far greater danger is also ever present; the possibility – really the probability – or rupture from any sudden strain.

A brief description of these muscles will enable you to understand more clearly the following exercise, designed for strengthening these muscles.

The external, or descending, oblique muscles are situated on the side and fore-part of the abdomen. They are the largest and most superficial of the broad, thin, flat muscles that brace and support the lower part of the abdomen. They are firmly attached to the external surface and lower borders of the inferior, or lower, ribs. From these cartilaginous attachments other smaller muscles proceed in various directions. They lap, overlap, and interlace, and thus form a muscular webbing designed to support and protect the underlying bowels and organs. These external muscles are again braced by a system of deep-seated internal muscles, the whole forming a wonderfully ingenious structure designed to support and protect the underlying organs.

At this part of the body great muscular strength is requisite to sustain the pressure of the viscera within. If these muscles become weakened, serious results may follow.

The importance of especially exercising and strengthening these supporting muscles is therefore evident. This is very difficult to accomplish when standing erect, but can be readily effected in a recumbent position, as follows:

Lying upon your back, as shown in the illustration below, bend one knee upwards and inwards; as you do so, draw up the hip of that side. You will find this action tenses all of the lower abdominal muscles. Then drop that leg back to its original position, and bend the knee, and draw up the hip of the other side.

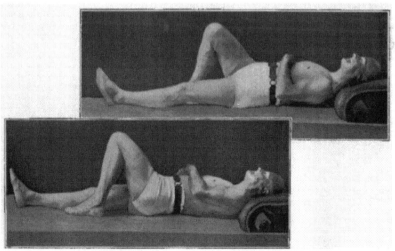

Developing the Lower Abdominal Muscles

Alternate in the exercising, first upon the right side, then the left.

The illustration shows the knee bent more than may be necessary, as after a few trials you will acquire control of the hip movement, after which the exercise will be very easy and improvement rapid.

Commence with three movements upon each side, increasing, as your physical condition in prove, to twenty-five.

This exercise is valuable in cases of constipation; and when the muscles described are toned up and strengthened, rupture is a very remote possibility.

Exercise for Strengthening the Loins
XV.

All of these exercises are perform in bed, under cover of the bed clothes

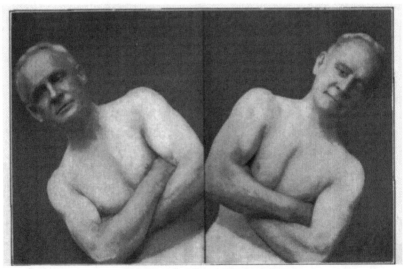

Developing the Loin Muscles

Exercise for Strengthening the Loins

In that system of military drill familiarly known as the "setting-up drill", there is an exercise especially designed for the development of the loins and side muscles. Standing erect, with the hands upon the hips, the men bend the upper part of the body as far to one side as possible; then reverse, bending to the other side, thus alternately tensing and relaxing the muscles of the loins. It is an excellent method of strengthening the body at the point, as well as a remedy for constipation.

This exercise can be easily performed while lying in bed.

Resting upon your back, with your arms folded across the chest, raise the head and shoulders slightly, so as to clear the pillow.

Commence with then movements; that is, five upon each side; as your physical condition improves, increase to twenty-five.

This action will tense the abdominal muscles, and place a moderate tension upon the loin muscles, the weight of the head and shoulders being as excellent substitute for the mechanical appliances sometimes used. I combination with, and following, the exercise with the lifting board, every muscle of the loins and sides will be brought into healthy action. If faithfully and systematically practiced, improvement is certain.

Exercise for the Development of the Legs
the climbing Muscles
XVI.

**All of these exercises are perform in bed,
under cover of the bed clothes**

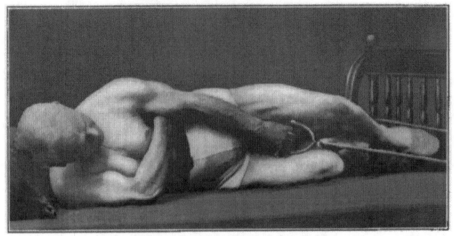

Developing the "Climbing Muscles"

Exercise for the Development
of the Legs
The Climbing Muscles

In most persons the legs, as they are constantly exercised in the ordinary pursuits of life, are proportionately better developed than the arms. But the mere exercise of walking will not specially develop the large muscles at the front of the thighs and in the calves of the legs, which I will designate as the "climbing muscles." Walking or running, while either brings those muscles into action, does not place any considerable tension upon them, and as a rule neither pedestrians nor fast runners are notable for any unusual development at these points;

while, on the other hand, bicyclists and "men of the hills" are almost invariably well developed there.

The leg muscles of the runner are more elastic, and capable of more rapid action, than are those of the adept of the silent wheel or the athlete of the hills, but the former soon tires under the strain of a steady climb, whatever his physical condition may be, simply because he has not developed the muscles then called into action.

It is really only a matter of training. My attention was called to this marked deficiency in the cases of several well-known runners and pedestrians, members of a celebrated San Francisco athletic club. Upon several occasions these gentlemen were the guests of an outing club to which I belonged for several years. We owned a small pack of fox hounds with which we were in the habit of hunting coyotes. The country in which we hunted in very rough, hilly, and impracticable for horses; we therefore followed the hounds on foot.

A coyote, when chased by hounds, always selects for his line of flight the roughest country he can find; and to cut off his flight usually meant a running climb over hills too steep and high to be available for anything but pasturage for the half-wild cattle wandering over them. If the run led up a valley or over level country our guests had not trouble in jogging on ahead of us, apparently a tireless as the hounds whose wild chorus echoed through the canyon; but when the scrub wolf changed his course, and started over the "high divide," the conditions changed. The elastic muscles of the athletes, accustomed only to the smooth floor of the gymnasium or the level cinder path, quickly tired when called upon to face the steep sides of "rocky ridge."

I have seen one of these gentlemen make a good showing in a five-mile flat race, while another once held a low mark at 220 yards, and at the time in question both were in excellent condition. But the steep grade and the steady strain of the "high divide," while but a jog for the slower men who were accustomed to the climb, were too much for them.

This, or any other athletic feat, is not so much a matter of natural ability, as of the training of the muscles specially brought into play by the exertion.

The development of these "climbing muscles" of the legs for any exercise of this nature will interest very few, but as a means of developing and adding that the simple and effective means I will suggest may be of more general interest. To bring into action the large muscles on the front of the thigh and those that make up the calf of the leg. *i.e.,* the "climbing muscles." it is necessary to exert a pressure upon the ball of the foot, which can be accomplished very easily as you lie in bed.

Attach to the foot of your bed a cord about 1½ feet in length, terminating in a pulley-weight handle. Lying upon your side, grasp this handle, then press firmly against the foot-board of the bed with the ball of the foot, and alternately relax the pressure. This alternate pressure and relaxation will actively exercise the muscles in question, will imitate the action of climbing with the leg so exercised, and will bring no strain or possible injury upon the heart – a danger ever imminent in hill climbing.

The pressure exerted should be equal to that required in climbing stairs or a steep grade. This exercise, if persistently and regularly practiced, will surely improve the symmetry of the legs, and will give one an ability to ascent stairs or climb steep hills, which can never be acquired by the same amount of walking or ordinary gymnasium running exercise. It should be practiced upon both the left and the right side; otherwise the development will be unequal.

Dyspepsia
XVII.

All of these exercises are perform in bed,
under cover of the bed clothes

Dyspepsia

Most people are afflicted with some form of digestive disorder, the "quick lunch habit" of the modern business man being more largely responsible for this condition than anything else; for it is not so much what you eat, as how you eat it. If you food is not thoroughly chewed, and, in that process, thorough in salivated, it will certainly be digested with difficulty when it reaches the stomach; and if this habit of swallowing the food hastily, and without proper mastication, is persisted in dyspepsia, with its various complications, will surely result.

There is no exception. Nature is a stern creditor, resenting any infraction of her laws. If you violate them, you will certainly suffer for it. And the severest penalties she inflicts are for transgressing the laws of digestion. Under the familiar title, dyspepsia, we group various distressing digestive disorders, most of which could be avoided by properly chewing the food.

I have stated that, in my personal experience, and by the system of exercises I practice, I have found it to be possible to build up the aged human body after it has passed the half-century limit, and to restore to it the muscular development it may have possessed in earlier years; and that it is also possible to excel that condition. But this cannot be done when serious digestive disorders exist; until they are remedied improvement will be slow. As the trouble is usually caused by hurried eating and, consequently, insufficient mastication, the logical remedy is to take more time at meals, and chew the food thoroughly. This change in habits alone will, most probably, greatly improve the digestive conditions in a short time.

The next step is to strengthen the muscles of the stomach, for the digestion of food depends largely upon the strength of those muscles.

In the process of digestion, the muscles of the stomach alternately contract and relax, producing a churning motion which, with the aid of the digestive fluids, digests the food. Now, if those muscles are weak, the work of digestion will be carried on poorly and with great effort. If this process of digestion were solely the result of chemical action, then a healthy condition might, possibly, be artificially brought about by medicinal preparations and cures might be effected by some of the numerous dyspepsia "dopes" advertised throughout the world. But, as muscular strength cannot be obtained from any drug, it is certain that these preparations cannot be the infallible remedies for digestive disorders the inventors and their advertisements claim for them. Temporary relief from the distress of indigestion may undoubtedly be obtained from these alleged remedies, and a more careful attention to diet – which the sufferer would most probably observe when taking them – would result in some improvement; but as will expect a cure by the use of opium, or any other anodyne, as to place dependence solely upon any drug, or combination of drugs.

The remedy lies with one's self, and, if the following brief directions are followed faithfully and persistently, any one will succeed as I have done.

Chew your food slowly, that it may be thoroughly in salivated and digested readily. It is also necessary to strengthen the muscles of the stomach. This can be accomplished by the following simple and easily-performed exercise:

Lying on your back, bend your head well forward. (This action will contract and tense the abdominal muscles.) When the head is dropped back to the horizontal position, those muscles will relax.

These alternate contraction and relaxation exercises will, of themselves, materially strengthen the muscles; but percussion will greatly aid in producing that result. Therefore, as you alternately raise and lower the head, and thus contract and relax the muscles, strike the abdomen rapidly with your clenched fists, at first lightly, but afterwards increasing the force of the blow, as the muscles become stronger. This exercise will determine the blood to that part, will produce a healthy circulation, and strengthen the digestive organs.

Another excellent exercise is to place the palms of the hands firmly upon the abdomen and rub back and forth, much in the way a washboard is used. These two exercises will also reduce any fatty deposit which may have accumulated, and are harmless, inexpensive, and far more effective than the most widely advertised and most lauded "dyspepsia cures."

I speak from experience, as I suffered from dyspepsia for over thirty years, vainly seeking relief during all that time, from the various medicinal remedies prescribed by physicians, or others which I was induced to purchase by advertisement or by the recommendation of sympathetic friends.

The causes of my trouble were hurried meals, insufficient mastication, and weakness of the abdominal muscles. My cure was effected by the system I have described. To those unfortunates who are afflicted as I have been, I strongly urge the practice of these exercises for strengthening the abdominal muscles.

Percussion Exercise for Strengthening the Abdominal Muscles and Improving Digestion
XVIII.

**All of these exercises are perform in bed,
under cover of the bed clothes**

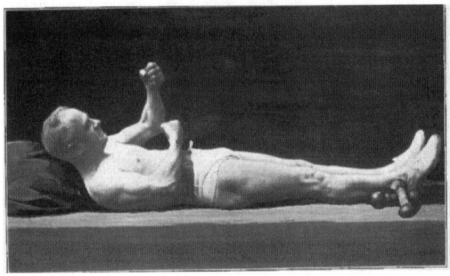

Developing the Abdominal Muscles by Percussion

**Percussion Exercise for Strengthening
the Abdominal Muscles and
Improving Digestion**

This method of exercise is described in the pages headed "Dyspepsia." There is but little to add to that statement. Suffice it, then, to say that it is an excellent exercise, and has a very beneficial effect upon all the digestive organs.

Commence with twenty-five quick strokes; increase, as your physical condition will warrant, to one hundred or more. The percussion should be light and rapid.

Continue the percussion, both in the tensed and relaxed conditions of the abdominal muscles, as produced in the foregoing exercise; the tension and relaxation being caused by alternately raising and lowering the head, as in the illustration on the previous page.

During intervals of rest, if it is desired to reduce abdominal fat, massage and rub the fatty deposit as directed upon the page headed "Reducing an Obese Abdomen". I have been accustomed to extend the body at full length in this exercise, as shown in the illustration; but if you find you are impeded by the bed clothes, bend the knees, which will raise the covering clear of the abdomen.

I strongly recommend this exercise to those suffering from indigestion.

The Reduction of an Obese Abdomen
XIX.

**All of these exercises are perform in bed,
under cover of the bed clothes**

The Reduction of an Obese Abdomen

Fat has been termed the packing of the body; and, while it is necessary to have sufficient of that packing to full up the interstices of the muscles, thus presenting the roundness of the body and limbs characteristic of health and youth, an excess is undesirable and frequently becomes a very serious affliction. Where there is a tendency to "take on fat" it is usually deposited in greater quantities upon the abdomen than upon any other part of the body, for the reason that the fat, being inert tissue, naturally gravitates to the point of least activity. The legs, arms, and back, being constantly exercised in the ordinary habits of life, do not offer such a favorable resting place for fat as the abdomen, upon which the deposit will first appear; consequently, in persons of sedentary habits, we frequently find attenuated limbs in marked contrast to an obese abdomen.

To remedy this unsatisfactory condition, various methods of diet are practiced. Of these the well-known systems of Banting and Schwenninger are probably the best. They are published in book form, and anyone interested can obtain them at most book stores. In many cases of corpulence the practice of these methods of diet, if adhered to persistently, will finally effect the desired result; but the danger in them is that the reduction of the system in general often produces a weakened condition which effects the heart. Added to this, the reduction of the fatty tissue, being general, is not especially directed to any particular part of the body, and the discomfort entailed in the practice of the systems does not invite its universal adoption. Furthermore, they involve a great deal of self denial.

My experience is that the method I practice and describe, in the following pages, is more effective, less troublesome, and without danger.

It is not definitely known what fat really is, or what is its cause. A carbohydrate diet, that is, such as contains starch or sugar in some form, usually produces the trouble; but, when the system has a well-defined tendency to form fat in excess of its normal condition, a course of dieting and attendant self-denial may not always be successful. We frequently hear corpulent people complain that "everything they eat turns to fat", which in a great measure often appears to be true.

Fat would seem to be undeveloped tissue, formed in the

ordinary process of digestion and assimilation, but upon reaching a certain stage is arrested in its further development, and, instead of becoming living cellular tissue, changes to this inert substance known to physiology as adipose tissue, or fat. When, from some unknown cause, an abnormal tendency has developed, causing an oversupply of this form of tissue, it is doubtful if the remedy lies alone in diet.

Muscular activity and agitation at the point of excessive deposit is probably the most direct, surest, easiest, and safest method of its elimination. This activity has the same effect upon such deposits as it has upon worn-out and clogging dead tissue, which I have explained can be forced from the point of lodgment by the alternate contraction and relaxation of the muscles. In short, by the exercise I practice and have described, fatty tissue, when thus dislodged, is carried off by the ordinary process of excretion; and my experience has been that, under no circumstances, is it possible to convert it into muscular tissue.

Obesity is evidently caused by local inactivity, and that being the case, the only logical and successful remedy would seem to be muscular activity or agitation, where the fatty deposit is situated. Walking is highly recommended and is undoubtedly beneficial; but it is only an indirect means of attacking the trouble, the motion of the legs not especially bringing into action the muscles of the abdomen, which are covered by the fatty deposit. Therefore, some more direct means of forcing into activity, and thereby dislodging this accumulation of inert adipose tissue, would be more effective. It is a logical deduction that, if the fat is accumulated by reason of sluggish surroundings, then any method which changes that condition to one of activity, will remedy the trouble.

The method I have found most effectual is massage while the abdominal muscles are tensed. The process will be more readily comprehended by full instructions.

Exercise for the Reduction of an Obese Abdomen
XX.

All of these exercises are perform in bed, under cover of the bed clothes

Exercises for the Reduction of an Obese Abdomen

Tense the muscles of the abdomen; place the palms of the hands upon it; pres down firmly; and rub the accumulation of fat back and forth, not permitting the hands to slip. Otherwise the skin only will be rubbed, and so benefit results.

Vary this process by striking the abdomen rapidly with your clenched fists, alternately contracting and relaxing the abdominal muscles. The act of contracting is easily accomplished by raising the head.

These exercises are a very effective method of attacking the objectionable despite, and if systematically and persistently practiced, will certainly achieve satisfactory results. Both of these exercises can be performed most easily and effectively in a recumbent position in bed.

Why adipose tissue disappears under this treatment is not altogether clear, but is certainly does.

Exercises for Developing the Muscles Covering the Shoulder Blades
XXI.

All of these exercises are perform in bed, under cover of the bed clothes

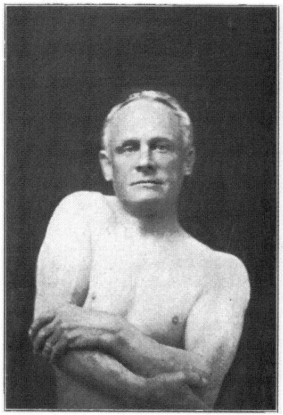

Developing the Muscles of the Shoulder Blades

Exercise for Developing the Muscles
Covering the Shoulder Blades

Lying upon your back, alternately raise your shoulders, as shown in the illustration on the opposite page. The tension should be upward and forward as far as possible.

Commence with five movements upon each side; it is perfectly safe, and in a very short time all feeling of soreness, which may result from the first attempts, will disappear. The movements can then be increased without fatigue, and with very satisfactory result to ten times the original number.

By reference to the anatomical plate facing page 29, you will see that this movement will bring into action the large muscles attached to, and covering, the shoulder blades. It is an excellent exercise for ladies who may be deficient at this point, improvement being certain if these directions are faithfully followed. If your shoulders were ever well developed and symmetrical, that condition can certainly be restored by persistent practice of this exercise.

Exercises for Broadening the Shoulders
XXII.

All of these exercises are perform in bed,
under cover of the bed clothes

Exercise for Broadening the Shoulders

Lying upon your back, grasp the left elbow with the right hand, and the right elbow with the left hands. (As pressure is exerted, you will feel an outward or lateral strain upon both shoulders.) The upper arms, under this cross pull, act as levers forcing them apart; the pressure from the right hand upon the left elbow acts upon the shoulders muscles of the left side, while a corresponding effect takes place upon the opposite shoulder. In this position, practice that motion familiarly known as shrugging the shoulders; the lateral strain the tensed condition of the muscles, combined with the up and down movement of the shoulders, is a most effective method of developing that part of the body.

Commence with five movements, increasing daily, as your strength and physical condition will warrant, until you have reached twenty-five with ease, and without any feeling of soreness. This is a very good and effective exercise, and will surely have the desired result if persistently practiced.

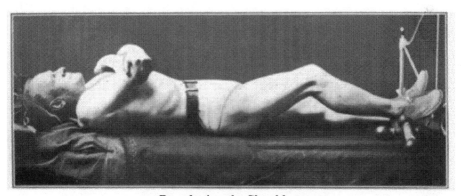

Broadening the Shoulders

The Lifting Board
XXIII.

All of these exercises are perform in bed,
under cover of the bed clothes

The Lifting Board

This simple but very effective device for exercising the muscles of the shoulders and loins and thighs is a board 15 inches in length, by

4 inches in width. At each end are inserted two strong screw eyes to which are attached ropes 18 inches long, terminating in ordinary pulley-weight handles. This board is covered with flannel, to prevent a chill to the feet.

The method of its use is shown by the illustration upon this page; the effect is that of the ordinary lifting machine, with the advantage that it is used in a recumbent position, and under cover of the bed clothes. It is the only exercise I practice in which there is any danger of injury, as it is possible to strain the muscles of the loins or shoulders, if too great force is exerted; therefore, in commencing the practice, put on the strain gently for a few seconds; then relax. This alternate tension and relaxation by the lifting movement specially brings into action the muscles of the shoulders, loins, and thighs; but it is also an excellent exercise for the whole body.

The apparatus is very simple and easily made. Do not use springs or elastic bands, which you will be tempted to do, thinking they are an improvement. I used them and abandoned them in favor of the inflexible ropes.

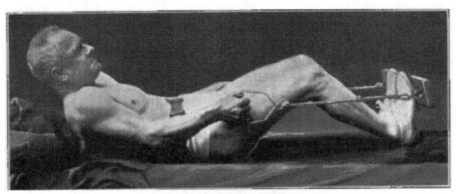

Using the Lifting Board

The elasticity of the loin muscles in the act of lifting will be sufficient, and you will be better able to determine the amount of lifting strain required. I strongly advocate this exercise, but in moderation. Commence with five gentle movements, increasing, as strength develops, and your physical condition may warrant.

Exercise for Developing and Strengthening the Neck
XXIV.

All of these exercises are perform in bed, under cover of the bed clothes

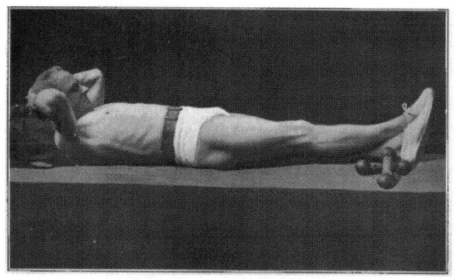

Developing the Muscles of the Neck

Exercise for Developing and Strengthening the Neck

Clasp the hands firmly back of the head, as shown in the illustration above. Raise the head clear of the pillow; then press it backward, exerting at the same time a strong forward, or resistance, pressure with the arms. Commence with not more than five movements; that is, alternately raising and lowering the head, at the same time keeping up the full strain of the arms. At the end of a week increase one or two movements, as your condition may warrant. My own limit is now twenty-five, which I find ample. By an excess of this exercise, I increased my neck measurement from fourteen to sixteen inches; which, being out of proportion to my height, I totally discontinued for about six months, the same measurement reducing to fifteen and one-quarter inches; at which it remains.

The muscles called into action, and specially developed by this exercise, are shown in the illustration facing page 29.

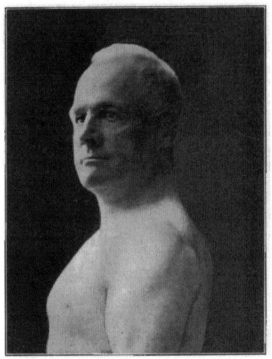

Developing of Throat Muscles

Stretching-Board Device for Broadening the Shoulders XXV.

All of these exercises are perform in bed, under cover of the bed clothes

Stretching-Board Device for Broadening the Shoulders

In most gymnasium there is an excellent exercised practiced to broaden the shoulders by the means of lateral tension. Standing between two upright parallel bars, the student grasps them with both hands, his arms outstretched at right angles to the body. The exercise consists in pulling alternately with either hand, first right, then left. This action exercises or stretches laterally the muscles of the shoulders, and, if regularly and persistently practiced, improvement is certain.

At the commencement of my efforts to devise simple methods of exercising in bed, as a substitute for the regular gymnasium exercise, I unsuccessfully experimented with rings, bars, and ropes, which I attached to the sides of the bed, endeavoring the effect lateral tension of the shoulder muscles by such means. I found that, in addition to the inconvenience of the fixtures, the body was unpleasantly shifted from side to side by the force of the pull; while the desired result, directly contrary to that, was an alternate tension and relaxation of the shoulder muscles, without any change in the position of the body.

Finally I tried a board, as long as the spread of my outstretched arms, and three inches in width. This I grasped at the ends, the pull of the opposing hands giving the lateral tension of the shoulder muscles without disturbing the position of the body. I found this stretching-board very effective, and the only improvement I have ever made upon it is to attach strong iron handles to the ends, that the hands may have a firmer and more convenient hold.

The Exercise is This:

Lying upon your back, with the board resting diagonally across the chest, the hands grasping the ends or handles, as in the illustration below, pull with your full force upward as far as possible, that the muscles under the arms and extending along the upper ribs may receive the strain; resist with a downward pull of equal force; next reverse the pull, that each side may be exercised.

Second Movement:

With the board lying at right angles across the chest, pull with both hands at once, keeping upthe strain for two or three seconds; then relax. Commence with five movements for each exercise; that is, alternately tensing and relaxing the muscles, as described; increase to fifteen movements, as your physical condition my warrant.

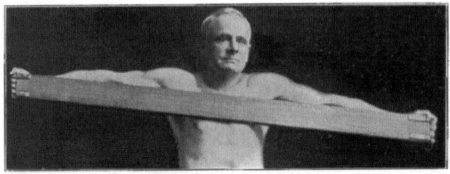

Using the Stretching Board

Dumb-Bell Exercise
In combination with Massage of the Biceps and Triceps Muscles
XXVI.

**All of these exercises are perform in bed,
under cover of the bed clothes**

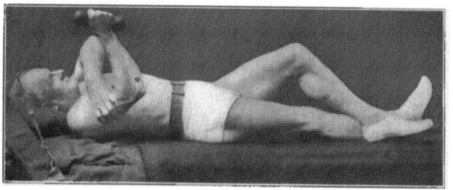

Developing the Arms by Dumb-Bell Exercise and Massage

Dumb-Bell Exercise

In Combination with Massage of the Biceps and Triceps Muscles

Development of the arms, by this method of exercise, is very much more rapid than by boxing, or any gymnasium exercise practiced with the usual mechanical appliances.

To the celebrated athletic, C.A. Sampson, one of the world's strong men and the rival of Sandow, seems due the credit of discovering that massage of the muscles during exercise greatly aids their development. The method employed by him was the application of strong elastic bands or straps, which he fastened tightly around his arms during his dumb-bell exercise. The alternate pressure and relaxation of the bands or straps, as the muscles were contracted or relaxed, made a very effective massage. He attributed his marvelous strength to this practice.

After studying his method, and the very logical reasons he advances in his book, "Strength," I procured the elastic straps described, and practiced according to his directions. The improvement that resulted was soon apparent, and it was evident that the system would effect all that its author claimed for it, but the inconvenience of the device was such that I abandoned it. I substituted the exercise shown on the opposite page, using, instead of the elastic straps or bands, simply the pressure of the hands clasped firmly over the upper arms, which I massage while I am suing the dumb-bell.

Development of the biceps and triceps muscles will be found to be very rapid by this system.

Commence practice with not more than ten movements; then increase gradually to fifty for each arm; this, with daily practice, should be sufficient to keep the arms strong and flexible. Weight of dumb-bells two to four pounds in accordance with your strength.

Dumb-Bell Exercise
XXVII.

All of these exercises are perform in bed, under cover of the bed clothes

Dumb-Bell Exercise for Two Hands

I strongly advocate the use of light dumb-bells. The pair I use weigh four pounds, but half that weight, in most cases, will be sufficient. I have experimented, as I lay in bed, with all sizes up to forty pounds, but I have found that moderately quick action with weights of from two to four pounds the most effective. There is always a danger of over exercise with the heavy dumbbells; the continuous strain may affect the heart, and certainly has a tendency to bring on that condition known in athletics as being "muscles bound."

The light weights with rapid action, in the position shown by the illustration upon this page, will give an elasticity and general quickness of motion which cannot be obtained with the heavy dumb-bells.

Commence with ten strokes; increase, as your condition will warrant, to fifty or more. It is a safe and effective and effective exercise. After this striking exercise is completed, extend your arms to their full length at right angles with the sides, and alternately turn, or twist, your wrists back and forth, so that the arms will partially revolve in their shoulder sockets. If there is any tendency to rheumatic pains at this point, where deposits of uric acid frequently occur, this movement will be found to be beneficial, as it will dislodge such deposits.

Commence with five movements and gradually increase to twenty-five, which at all stages will be sufficient.

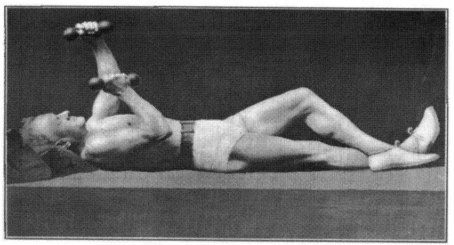

Developing the Arms by Dumb-Bells Exercise

The Liver
XXVIII.

**All of these exercises are perform in bed,
under cover of the bed clothes**

The Liver

When the liver is wrong everything seems wrong everything seems wrong, for the health of the body depends largely upon its condition and activity. If it secretes bile normally, and performs its other functions healthfully, then the whole body has the benefit of its good work; but if, on the other hand, it is lazy congested, troubles commence; a torpid or fractious liver being a very serious affliction. The list of troubles resultant from this condition is a long one.

The liver is really a filter through which the blood must pass to be purified, and if this process of purification is improperly performed the blood is poisoned, and any or all of the organs may be affected more or less seriously. When the liver is sluggish there is usually a dull, aching pain in the right side, and often under the right shoulder blade. Then, too, there are pains in the forehead, (more rarely in the back of the head); furred tongue; an unpleasant taste in the mouth at morning; a dingy, yellow color in the whites of the eyes; loss of appetite, and often dizziness; drowsiness after meals, and a generally pessimistic view of life. These are some of the disagreeable conditions that result, in varying degrees of intensity, and there are others more serious that may follow, if this, one of the most important organs of the human system, is not kept up to its normal activity.

Without going into the physiology details and functions of the liver, think of it simply as a filter through which the blood must pass to be freed from its impurities, and remember that it must be kept in an active state to properly perform its duties. To accomplish this it must be exercised, as must every other organ of the body, the simplest and most effective method being rhythmical agitation, or massage, performed by oneself in bed, preferably in the early morning, when the stomach is empty.

It is best to first acquaint yourself with the position, size, and general characteristics of the liver, before commencing the exercises that follow. The liver is a gland, or rather a multitude of glands, bound together in one conglomerate body. In an adult it usually weighs four pounds, and is nearly one foot in length in its longest dimensions. It is situated upon the right side of the body. It occupies a large space in the abdomen just under the diaphragm, and is partially covered by the lower ribs. The most accessible point for its exercise or agitation is immediately above the angle of the right hip bone, and under the lower ribs.

It is held firmly in place by five strong ligaments, and nothing but great abuse, such as tight lacing, unnatural pressure, or accidental injury to the region, can displace it; hence there is not possibility that the method of exercise I describe will injure the organ. After five years of practice I can confidently state that benefit alone will result, and that under the most comfortable conditions, and without medicine or expense.

The practice of the three exercise which follow, in combination with those previously described, with surely relieve you of the presence of that child of the Evil One – Liver Compliant – and its companion – Dyspepsia.

Exercising the Liver
XXIX.

**All of these exercises are perform in bed,
under cover of the bed clothes**

Exercising the Liver

First Exercise

Lying on your back, as shown in the illustration on the next page, place the ends of the fingers of both hands over that region of the liver at the right side of the abdomen, above the angle of the right hip bone, and below the edge of the lower rib. Then press the fingers upward and well under the rib. The abdominal muscles, being in a relaxed condition in this position, will readily yield to the pressure, and the liver can easily be move or agitated. Press under a upward, and then relax the pressure, commencing with twenty movements, and increasing up to one hundred when your condition will warrant.

The effect of this agitation of the organ is the same as that obtained in riding a trotting horse, an exercise universally recommended by physicians when the liver is sluggish.

Second Exercise

Lying upon your right side, place your left hand over the region of the liver previously described. Incline the head slightly forward and bend the knees, as shown in the illustration on the next page. (In this position the abdominal muscles will be relaxed and the liver inclined slightly forward.) Press either the ends of the fingers, or the knuckle of the thumb, well under the ribs, and massage, or agitate, the liver as in the preceding exercise.

While it is true that the first exercise may be sufficient, yet this change of position seems to present another surface for manipulation; and both positions can be practiced with good results.

Third Exercise (Percussion)

Percussion over the region of the liver will also promote its activity. The most advantageous position is upon the left side, the organ then being inclined slightly forward, and the muscles relaxed. Clench the right hand and strike lightly, but rapidly, at the point described.

Commence with twenty light blows, increasing the number to one hundred or more, as your condition will warrant.

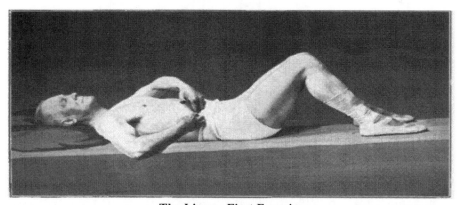

The Liver – First Exercise

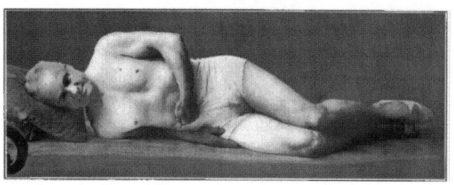

The Liver – Second Exercise

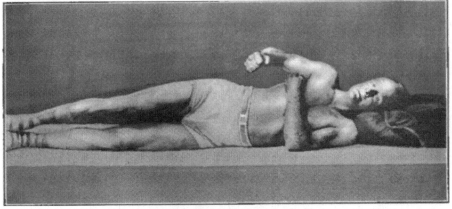

The Liver – Third Exercise

The Neck
XXX.

**All of these exercises are perform in bed,
under cover of the bed clothes**

The Neck

The principal supports of the neck are two large muscles attached to the base of the skull, and from thence descending to the shoulders;- they from the back of the neck. The sides are braced by another pair of large muscles which are attached to the skull immediately behind the ears, and which descend to the collar bone. These large muscles are braced by minor ones, but upon these main supports the contour and strength of the neck largely depend. If they are poorly developed the back and sides of the neck will appear weak and unsymmetrical; the skin-covering, lacking the proper support, will soon fall into unsightly creases; and in this condition there is an appearance of age which the time of life may not warrant.

Persistent rubbing of the back and sides of the neck with the palm of the hand will, to a considerable extent, efface these wrinkles; but this is a superficial treatment and its effect is but temporary; as, if the underlying muscles are shrunken and weak, the skin – being poorly supported – will surely become loose and flabby, and the creases will deepen.

The remedies dear to the feminine mind for this condition are so-called "skin foods" and other greasy preparations of like nature. But as it is impossible to form muscular tissue by their use, the fallacy of the process is evident. The skin will certainly be improved by the friction necessary to apply the preparations, but aside from this the treatment is of no avail.

It is evident that if the muscles described were developed and restored to the condition of earlier years, the skin, being then properly supported, would regain its smooth surface. This can be accomplished by the following exercise.

Exercising the Neck
XXXI.

All of these exercises are perform in bed,
under cover of the bed clothes

Exercising the Neck

Lying upon your side, as shown in the illustration on the opposite page, turn the chin as far as possible towards the upper shoulders. (This movement will contract the muscles upon the side of the neck, and will also bring into action those muscles of the throat immediately under the chin.) When the head drops back to its original position the muscles will relax. Their alternate contraction and relaxation an exercise which will develop the muscles of the sides of the neck, and will also strengthen and improve the contour of the throat muscle.

Commence the exercise with five movements, and increase to fifty or more, as your physical condition improves. Both sides of the neck must be exercised, for otherwise the development will be unequal.

The effect of this exercise upon the neck is shown in the illustration facing page 80. The deep lines which once crossed and re-crossed the back of my neck have wholly disappeared, and my appearance at the point is that of a man of half my years.

Ladies who may contemplate practicing this exercise need not fare the appearance of undue muscularity which this picture exhibits. The effect of exercise upon the muscles of women is not the same as upon the muscles of men. The knotted and rugged appearance of the muscles of the trained male athlete never appear in women, although similarly trained. Their muscles always remain soft, elastic, and more graceful in their roundness than those of men.

The exercise here described will improve and beautify the neck at a time when, in middle life, it is usually very scrawny.

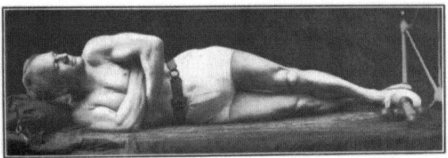

Developing the Muscles of the Neck

The Muscles of the Throat
XXXII.

**All of these exercises are perform in bed,
under cover of the bed clothes**

The Muscles of the Throat

These are voluntary muscles and can be exercised at will. They can be increased in size. They can be increased in size, strength, and elasticity. The anatomical illustrations facing page 86 and 89, accurately define the appearance and position of these muscles. Upon them the contour of the throat largely depends. In the illustration facing page 86 you will notice a large muscles attached to that projection in (more familiarly, Adam's Apple), and form that point ascending to the lower part of the chin, where it is attached. It youth that muscles is usually full, round, and elastic, supporting the surrounding tissue and covering skin, filling up the hollows, and giving to the throat the roundness and graceful contour of the which the illustration facing page 181 is an excellent example.

As years creep on, if that part of the throat is not exercised, this large muscles, and the minor ones surrounding it, following the general law, deteriorate in strength, elasticity, and size; the tissue shrinks, and skin, without its former support, becomes seamed and wrinkled; then, later, falls into loose hanging folds, - the throat of old age. (See illustration facing page 84). If the muscles underlying the loose-hanging skin, as shown in this picture, could be brought back to their former size and condition, it is evident that the contour of the throat would be greatly improved, for it would assume the outline of earlier years. At what age this improvement, by the methods I practice, becomes impossible, I am unable to say. The photograph which faces page 20 was taken when I was entering my fiftieth year; it shows, under the chin, the loose-hanging skin of age, and that condition remained until I had entered my sixtieth year.

During the period of that ten years. I had industriously and successfully endeavored to improve the rest of my body, but had neglected to exercise the muscles of the throat and face, which consequently presented signs of physical age, in marked contrast to the more youthful appearance of the body and limbs. It being evident that this deterioration was due to the inactivity of these muscles, I devised a system of exercises for their development.

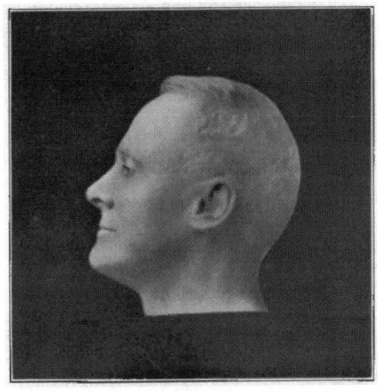

The Result of Throat Exercise

EXERCISING IN BED

The results of two years persistent practice in this direction are shown in the profile picture facing page 80. The throat muscles have regained their former strength and roundness, and the skin, being well supported, has caused the loose folds, which are shown in the photograph taken sixteen years ago, to disappear. There is a remarkable improvement over the conditions which then existed. This development of the throat, as well as of the entire neck, has been accomplished with much less exertion, and in less time, than was required to develop the arms and the legs. The most probable reason is, that the throat and face muscles, having never been exercised to any extent, were consequently must atrophied; and this improvement, when they were systematically exercised, was more noticeable. With my personal experience in this direction, I feel warranted in stating that it is possible, and really not difficult, to develop the muscles of the throat and face, by the methods described, after middle age; even after the half-century mark has been passed, wrinkles will disappear, and much of the smoothness of skin characteristic of earlier years may be regained. In short, if you will systematically and persistently practice the methods I have endeavored to make clear, the face and neck will assume a much more youthful appearance.

This will require some exertion upon your part, and some time; but it cannot be accomplished in any other way, all statements of the manufacturer and seller of "skin foods," face ointments, or any rejuvenating preparations, to the contrary. I speak from experience, as I experimented systematically and persistently with various "skin foods" and facial ointments for one year, feeling sure that if I could find any preparation which could be forced through the pores of the skin, and absorbed by the underlying glands, it might be possible to resore to the shrunken muscles of the face and throat the condition of earlier years. The result of that year of experiments was a complete failure, for the reason that the cellular tissue of which these muscles, as well as every other muscles and organ of the body is formed, is the result of the digestion and assimilation of the food we take into our stomachs, the fluids we drink, and the air we breathe. It is impossible to feed or nourish the muscles by any artificial means ever discovered. These so-called "skin foods" or face creams are not absorbed to any appreciable extent, and the improved appearance of the skin after their application is due to the pores of the skin and the myriads of small lines becoming temporarily filled up with the greasy preparation, while the smooth surface is due to the rubbing necessary to apply it. As before stated, the skin, like any other piece of leather, will polish much better with the palms of the hands dray and clean, than if coated with any greasy mixture.

There is no royal road to health; it cannot be bought; and if you have ever been endowed with physical beauty, don't waste your time and your money endeavoring to regain it by purchase, for that is not possible.

The rejuvenating methods I have described entail no expense or pain. They are very effective, but their practice rests with you, yourself, and they require both time and patience. If you value your personal appearance sufficiently to work for its improvement systematically and with persistence upon the lines described, my experience is that you will surely succeed. If, however, you conclude, as many will, that it is too much trouble, cultivate a spirit of contentment with your lot, and become resigned to the wrinkles and other indications of physical age, as it is impossible to remove them in any other way than as I have described.

Exercise for the Development of the Throat Muscles

First Exercise

XXXIII.

All of these exercises are perform in bed, under cover of the bed clothes

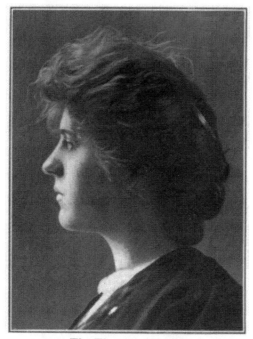

The Throat of Youth

Exercise for the Development of the Throat Muscles

First Exercise

Lying upon your side, place your thumb on the throat immediately under the chin, or at about the center of the large muscle which extends from the Adam's Apple to the chin (see anatomical plate facing page 89). If you lie upon your right side, use the right thumb; if upon the left, use the left thumb. Throw the head back to the position shown in the illustration on page 85.

Then bring the head forward (chin to the chest) which will relax the tension. Keep up the pressure of the thumb while alternating, contracting and relaxing the muscles by the movements described. This movement will tense the muscles of the throat, which the exercise is intended to develop, the firm upward pressure of the thumb and adding to that tension.

Commence with ten movements each morning, increasing gradually, as your physical condition will warrant, to fifty.

This exercise should be practiced while recumbent, both upon the right and left sides. If practiced faithfully and systematically a marked improvement of the contour for the throat will surely result.

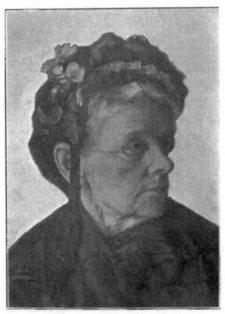

The Throat of Old Age

Exercise for the Development of the Throat Muscles
Second Exercise
XXXIV.

**All of these exercises are perform in bed,
under cover of the bed clothes**

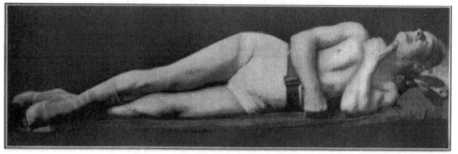

Developing the Throat Muscles

Exercise for the Development of the Throat Muscles

Second Exercise

In the same position of the body without any change in the point of thumb-pressure upon the throat muscles, turn the chin towards the upper shoulder as far as possible (as in the illustration above). This movement will tensed the large muscles at the side of the neck, as well as produce a lateral tension upon several of the small supporting muscles of the throat, which should also be exercised (anatomical plate, facing page 89.) The upward thumb-pressure will assist in the act of turning the chin toward the upper shoulders, and will add to the muscular tension produced by that movement. Relax the tension by turning the head back to the original position. Keep up the pressure of the thumb, while alternately contracting and relaxing the throat muscles, by the movements described.

Commence with ten movements, gradually increasing, as your physical condition will warrant, to fifty.

All of these exercises are designed for both the right and left sides, for if one side alone is exercised, development will be unequal. If there is any feeling of dizziness, practice only the first throat exercise.

The Rejuvenation of the Face and Neck XXXV.

All of these exercises are perform in bed, under cover of the bed clothes

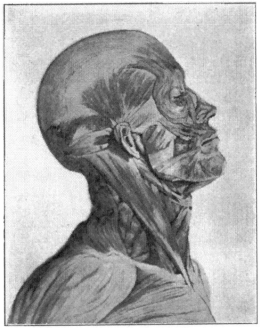

Muscles of the Throat – Head Thrown Back

The Rejuvenation of the Face and Neck

The exercise I have described, If persistently and methodically practiced, will surely restore to the an aged body mach of the lost strength and elasticity of an earlier period of life; for it is possible in this way to restore to the muscles of age the rounded contour they may have once possessed. But if the muscles, especially of the face and neck, are neglected they will present the relaxed and flabby condition characteristic of old age, even though the rest of the body has been developed to the strength of an athlete. The face and the neck, even while one is in vigorous training, may show the wear and deterioration of years, in marked contrast to the apparently more youthful body.

It is therefore necessary to exercise those muscles just as you have exercised the muscles of the body, and they will surely grow in size, strength, and elasticity if so trained. The hollow places in the neck and cheeks can be filled up, the muscles which surround the eyes can be increased in plumpness; and, with a treatment I will now describe, that smoothness of the skin characteristic of youth may, to a very considerable extent, be regained.

And this much-to-be-desired condition can be accomplished without cost and without the application of any "skin foods" or other nonsensical frippery of the kind. The process of digestion and assimilation alone can form the cellular tissue of which our bodies are built; and the lanoline, lard, paraffine, etc., which are usually the basis of these so-called "skin foods" are simply smeared on the skin and are not absorbed to any appreciable extent; nor can they be converted into cellular tissue by any amount of rubbing. The skin and muscles, absolutely, cannot be "fed" in that way or with such material, and any improvement in the appearance of the skin which seems to result from their use, is due solely to the friction required in applying the supposed palliative. If a face ointment is desired, use pure olive oil. It will soften the outer skin, is cleanly, and, well worked in, will be absorbed, to a limited extent; and, after being rubbed off, will leave the skin clear and soft.

The true secret of restoring to the skin the smoothness of youth if friction. The skin can be polished like any other leather, and the palms of the hands and tips of the fingers are the very best tools to use for that purpose.

This polishing can be best and most conveniently done as you lie in bed; and, again, like any other leather, the skin will polish much better dry than if moistened. Alternate the polishing process by slapping the face vigorously, thus accelerating the circulation and producing the healthy, ruddy glow of health. If the noise is objectionable, strike only with the fingers; the result will be the same.

The finer grades of soap do not injure the skin. In my morning ablutions I find the shaving soap used by barbers very satisfactory and far the best. S a lotion, after I have washed my face. I use borax, always keeping in a convenient place a quart bottle of water in which has been dissolved as large an amount of borax as the water will take up. I pour a couple of tablespoonfuls of this lotion into the wash basin, dilute it with a cupful of hot water, and bathe my face. There is a tonic effect in the borax which produces a smooth surface to the skin unequalled by any other lotion I know of. When the face is thoroughly dried, after the application, apply a few drops of purest olive oil; rub in well with the palms of the hands, and wipe dry with a soft bath towel. This treatment, if carefully and persistent followed, will greatly improve the texture of the skin, giving to the face and neck a fresh, healthy, and youthful appearance.

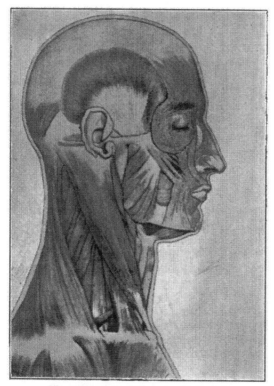

Muscles of the Throat – Relaxed

Exercises for the Development of the Face and Neck Muscles XXXVI.

**All of these exercises are perform in bed,
under cover of the bed clothes**

Exercises for the Development of the Face and Neck Muscles

The practice of the exercises especially designed for the development of the face and neck muscles require that you have a knowledge of their locations and uses. The anatomical plate facing this page will serve as a chart. You will notice that the eyes are surrounded by circular hands of muscles. In youth they were plump and sustained the overlying skin, keeping its surface smooth and unwrinkled; but, as years lapsed, they shrank in size, through lack of exercise, just as any other muscles of the body would deteriorate under like conditions. The skin covering them lost its support and fell into creases and lines, which we know as wrinkles – the certain indications of physical age. For those wrinkles there can be but one cure, and that is the restoration of their former plumpness to the supporting muscles. If this is not done all efforts towards the eradication of the disfiguring creases and lines will be futile.

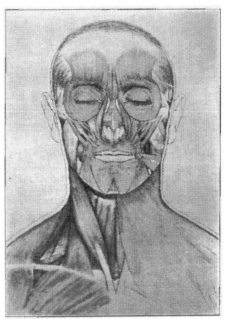

Muscles Surrounding the Eyes

The encircling eyes muscles may be classed as involuntary muscles, and cannot, to any beneficial effect, be controlled and exercised by the will.

Their development can only be accomplished by massage. To do this, use the heel of the hand, pressing it upon the bony structure immediately below, and at the corners of, the eyes, that it may rest upon the underlying muscles. Press firmly, that the hand may not slip, and practice the massage movement for several minutes.

Alternate this process by striking rapidly with the tips of the fingers. This percussion action is very beneficial, as it carried the blood to the part so treated, and is of great aid in the promotion of growth of tissue. If these exercises are persistently and systematically practiced, they will increase the shrunken muscles, even to plumpness and the skin, being supported as it was in youth, the crows feet and disfiguring wrinkles under the eyes will disappear.

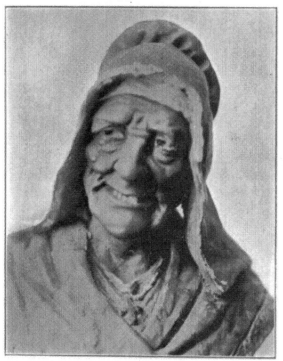

The Flabby Cheeks of Old Age

The Lines of Age
XXXVII.

**All of these exercises are perform in bed,
under cover of the bed clothes**

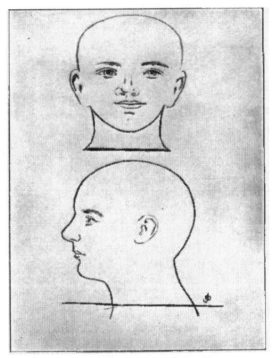

The Smooth Face of Youth

The Lines of Age

As we advance in years certain lines appear upon the face and neck which we associate with age; but these marks of physical deterioration are more often due to neglect than to years. In some women, for instance, they appear at twenty-five; in others, ten years later.

After persistent experiment upon the skin and muscles, for the past seventeen years, I am confident that if the practice of the simple methods described in this book are commenced when the disfiguring lines first appear, it is possible, not alone to efface them, but also to prevent their reappearance, until extreme old age.

The preservation of the celebrated Beauty of the Sixteenth Century, Ninon de Lenclos, is a well-known instance of this theory. This woman was remarkable for her wonderful physical preservation. Al the age of eighty, creditable authorities state, she retained the great beauty of her girlhood, her face having the freshness of youth, and being as free then from the lines of age as it had been at twenty, her while-powdered hair, then fashionable, but adding to her youthful appearance.

From the data the writer has been able to gather her smoothness of skin and freedom from wrinkles was due solely to persistent daily friction of the skin of her face, combined with an exercise for the muscles of the neck and throat, very similar to the exercises illustrated and described in this volume. Little was known of the laws of scientific physical culture at that time, but as Madam de Lenclos retained her elasticity of body and graceful figure to the last, it is evident that some system of exercises was systematically and persistently practiced. In that way alone could her youthful condition have been preserved.

Usually the first marks left by time upon the human features – and they are common to us all – are the wrinkles extending from the nostrils to the corners of the mouth, and beyond. As the years advance these are joined by parallel wrinkles, somewhat shorter, about half an inch distant on the cheek. Still later, another, and even shorter, wrinkle appears at a further distance of less than half an inch; and others are also formed, beginning at the corners of the mouth, and extending downward with a slight inward curve.

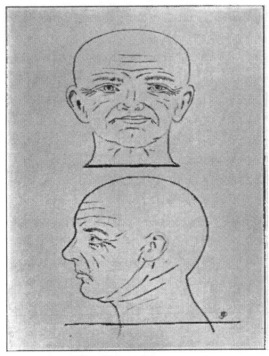

The Lines of Age

Wrinkles on the forehead which parallel the line of the eyebrows, with a slight downward bend at the ends, appear. These are generally from three to five in number, according to one's age. The wrinkles commonly called "crow's feet" spread, fanwise, from the outer corners of the eyes over the temples, and are usually from three to five in number.

The skin below the eyes becomes loose and creased. These creased lines start from the corners of the eyes, slightly curving, and overlapping each others. By this time one or two lines usually appear at the sides of the neck, commencing at a point back of the ears, extending below the jaw, and slanting downward to the throat. Immediately behind the ears, too, the skin becomes slightly loose; two short wrinkles from, and a line appears extending down to, and under, the neck. At the next stage a great number of very short, tiny lines begin to appear all over the face and neck – some parallel, others intersecting. These give to the skin a withered appearance. The freshness of youth has departed. Now, too, the skin under the chin becomes loose; all of the long lines meet and overlay and interweave, and combine with the short ones, just appearing, to form a tangled web of criss-crossings that deepen as the years advance. This is the skein of life. This is the spinning of time. And the pattern is never beautiful!

The only sure method of erasing these lines is by friction, and this is best accomplished with the dry palms of the hands, as described in the chapter upon the skin. This treatment, if commenced when disfiguring lines first appear, and if methodically and daily practiced, in combination with the exercise for the muscles of the face and neck, (described fully in the chapter upon that subject), will surely effect a very marked and satisfactory improvement in the personal appearance.

The Skin
XXXVIII.

All of these exercises are perform in bed, under cover of the bed clothes

The Skin

The skin forms a protective covering, a closefitting garment, for the whole body. It is of unequal thickness; over those parts which are exposed to pressure and friction it is thick and tough, but in the case of other parts liable to variations in size it is especially elastic. But in every place it is adapted to the purpose of protection.

It is both a secreting and an excreting organ, and upon its proper action our health, our very lives, depend. If its millions of glands and pores become obstructed it is impossible for one to be healthy. On the other hand, when these openings – the safety valves of the body – are free and clear, the impurities of the body are readily thrown off, the circulation is improved, an equilibrium is established in the eliminating process between the skin and the internal organs, digestion is easier, intestinal and urinary secretions become more regular, and an improvement in the nervous condition results. My own experience has been that daily friction of the skin with goat-hair mittens and a goat-hair friction belt will materially relive insomnia. These friction exercises should be followed by a tepid bath. The moral of it all is: Keep the skin clean by friction and bathing.

The skin is composed of three layers. Overlying the true skin is the cuticle, or scarf skin, and although we commonly call this the skin, it is really only a protecting layer over the true skin. It has no blood vessels, so it never bleeds; and, as it contains no nerves, it feels no pain. The microscope shows that it is composed entirely of minute flat scales which overlap each other very much like the shingles of a roof. These scales are formed by the true skin beneath, and are constantly thrown off from the body. Ordinarily this is imperceptible; but sometimes the scales accumulate into masses, when it is called scurf. Or, if the accumulation is upon the scalp, it is known as dandruff.

Upon the condition of the scarf skin the complexion largely depends. If it is rough, a good complexion is impossible. Temporary improvement can be obtained by use of the remedies dear to the feminine mind – "skin foods," face creams, and face powders. But all of these applications have the same result; they simply fill up the minute lines, and temporarily smoothe the rough surface. But when this coating is washed off, the skin will resume its former condition.

It is not usually claimed for face powders that they will afford more than a temporary improvement, but the manufacturers and venders of so called "skin foods" positively assert that their preparations feed and nourish the skin, and build up the underlying muscles, and that the benefit derived from their use is therefore permanent. If lanoline, paraffine, white wax, and spermaceti, the basis of all these preparations, could be forced into the true skin and the muscles, and could there converted into living cellular tissue, of which all parts of the body (the skin included) are composed, this claim might have some foundation of truth. But as these cells can only come into life by the process of digestion and assimilation, the fallacy of the above claim is apparent. You certainly cannot form or "build up" living tissue from dead matter. The term "skin food" is a very attractive title for these greasy, waxy preparations, but neither the skin nor the muscles can feed on that kind of food. By friction some slight absorption of the higher grades of oil is possible; but even this does not become living tissue. As this absorption is limited to only the very highest grades of oil, it is manifestly impossible for the skin to take up paraffine, while wax, or any of the other coarse concomitants of "skin foods."

Their immediate effect, as before stated, is to coat the surface of the skin, which, after their use, assumes a smoother appearance. But this is temporary, and there can be no growth or improvement of the underlying muscles by such applications. The objection to these greasy ointments is that they clog up and obstruct the myriads of underlying pores and glands. If you would have a healthy skin, these outlets for the impurities of the system must be kept clean and clear. Otherwise the skin cannot be healthy.

The secret of a fresh, healthy skin is friction and cleanliness. Upon the body use the goat-hair friction mittens and the friction belt of the same material. It is advisable that these friction exercises be practiced daily – after the other exercises described in this book – and followed by a tepid bath.

For the face and neck, friction with the dry palms of the hands in an effective method of removing wrinkles, as they can be rubbed out, and the skin can be polished, as elsewhere stated, just like any other piece of leather. For the ablutions of the face and neck use tepid water softened with borax, as already advised.

In a very short time after commencing these friction exercises for the body you will find that the nervous system is quieter and that both the digestion and the circulation are improved. And what will prove of special interest to ladies is that the friction exercises for the face and neck will surely result in a marked improvement.

I have demonstrated upon my own face and neck that by this method wrinkles can be removed even in advanced age, and I am position that if this friction exercise is commenced when the lines first appear and is persistently practiced, they will be eradicated and will not again appear until extreme old age. This is the method that was practiced by Ninon De Lenclos, the celebrated French beauty of the seventeenth century, and it is the only successful method for removing wrinkles and retaining the smooth skin characteristic of youth.

The Muscles of the Cheeks
XXXIX.

All of these exercises are perform in bed,
under cover of the bed clothes

The Muscles of the Cheeks

As years creep on the cheeks sink in and hollows appear in them where, once, they were full and plump. This is due to the shrinking of the supporting muscles, as shown in the illustration facing page 91.

There are four of these muscles on each side of the face; they are attached to the cheek bones under the eyes, and from thence descend, and are attached to the jaw. As we grow older, these muscles lose their strength and elasticity, and this change produces the pendant, or loose, jowl characteristic of age, just as their lessened size is the cause of the hollows in the cheeks. These are voluntary muscles, and can be exercised at will just as you would exercise the muscles of the arms or the legs.

Exercises for the Development of the Muscles Supporting the Cheeks
XL.

All of these exercises are perform in bed, under cover of the bed clothes

Exercises for the Development of the Muscles Supporting the Cheeks

First Exercise

Draw up the corner of the mouth towards the eyes, in the position of an exaggerated smile. In this contracted position press your fingers upon your cheeks, and you will find the muscles much thicker than when at rest.

Faithfully practice this movement, that is, alternately contracting and relaxing; and in a very short time the muscles will increase in size, and will fill up the hollows and restore to the cheeks the roundness of earlier years.

Second Exercise

In this exercise contract the muscles of the right side of the face, drawing the corner of the mouth as far toward the eye as possible; hold, in that position, for a few seconds; then change, repeating the process on the left side. Alternate this exercise with the first one described. It is not a valuable, but brings into action some minor muscles, which also require development.

These facial contortions present a somewhat comical and laughter-provoking appearance, but they are very effective; and I have not found any other exercise for the cheek muscles which show such satisfactory results. As they can be practiced in the privacy of your bedroom, comment need not be excited. Massage for the cheeks, as usually practiced while of some benefit, is far inferior to this method, for the reason that the cheek-supporting muscles are deep seated, and, lacking support, the rubbing or massaging process at this point is not very successful. The practice of rubbing "skin foods" or other ointments upon the cheeks in the hope that they will be absorbed, and thus build up the shrunken muscles and tissue, is a fallacy: upon this point, as I have previously commented, my experience is that the exercise I have described will, alone, achieve the desired result. I practice this alternate contraction and relaxation of the cheek muscles in connection with all of my bodily exercises, and it has become so much of a habit that it is performed unconsciously, and without effort or discomfort.

Massage for the Muscles of the Chin
XLI.

All of these exercises are perform in bed,
under cover of the bed clothes

Massage for the Muscles of the Chin

The muscles of the chin may be classed as involuntary, and can only be developed by massage; but they usually respond more quickly to that process than the muscles that surround the eye.

Rest the chin upon the palms of your hands; pres firmly; and rub the underlying muscles vigorously; the same method described for the muscles surrounding the eye, but requiring more pressure.

The position of the hands should be continually shifted, for, if continuous pressure is maintained upon any part without relaxation, growth is not so rapid. Change positions, as I have suggested, and if your chin was ever full and round in youth, that condition will, by persistent practice, be regained.

The Hair
XLII.

All of these exercises are perform in bed, under cover of the bed clothes

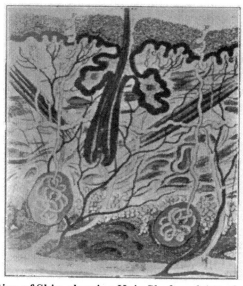

Cross Section of Skin, showing Hair-Shaft and Attached Muscles

The Hair

To understand the cause of the loss of hair and how to prevent that is fortune, it is necessary to know how the hair itself is formed, and how nourished, and the conditions favorable or unfavorable to its growth. Having learned this, the methods by which its loss can be arrested, and vitality regained, may be more readily comprehended and successfully practiced.

Facing page 101 appears an illustration which shows a transverse section of the skin of the scalp. This is taken from a greatly enlarged photograph, showing very clearly how the hair shaft, with its minute muscles and capillaries, appears under the microscope. The illustration exhibits a single hair; it is a tube composed of the same element as the nails or the bones. The secretions by which all three are formed are the same, and they do not appear to decrease as age advances. Therefore the immediate cause of the loss of hair would seem to be, and usually is, local. Tight or heavy hats, dissipation, sexual excesses, weakness of the muscles which are attached to each root of hair, defective circulation, uncleanliness of the scalp, microbes or germ diseases in the scalp, and failure to remove dead hairs which impede the growth of new ones; any of these may produce baldness. Remove the cause, or causes; follow the simple directions contained in this chapter; and wherever life remains in the follicles, or hair roots, new hairs will sprout. But if life has departed from them no power on earth can grow hair.

If the trouble is constitutional, or from any cause which tends to lessen the vital forces, practice the simple system of physical culture I have already described.

The result will surely be an improvement in the general physical condition, and a proportionate improvement in the health of the hair.

The coloring matter is negated in the hair bulb, and from there forced up through the tubular hair shaft. The character of the secretions determines the color of the hair. What the chemical combinations which produce that color are, we do not know; but as years increase, there is evidently a chemical change in the secretions, which causes a loss of the coloring matter. My own experience, and the result of sixteen years research, in this direction is that is not possible to restore the color when it has once departed, all of the preparations advertised for that purpose, with the thousands of testimonials to their infallibility, to the contrary. I will modify that statement: you can restore it with dyes, but the deception is sure to be detected sooner or later, and, added to this, the dye will injure the hair.

The scalp is similar to the face or any other part of the body. It is filled with thousands of little pores, which are constantly eliminating refuse matter; in addition to which the sebaceous glands throw off a certain amount of oil which adheres to the scalp. This dirt and animal fifth must be removed, or the pores will be clogged, - a condition which is very injurious.

When the hair is long, as usually worn by women, the scalp should be thoroughly cleaned at least twice a month; or, if of the ordinary length worn by men, at least twice a week. The best soap for the purpose is that used by barbers for shaving, as it seems least injurious to the skin.

Don't be afraid of water and good soap. Thousands lose their hair through neglecting to shampoo it properly. On the other hand, it is doubtful if any injury can result by the opposite extreme, provided the hair is thoroughly dried after the cleansing process. When dry, a few drops of olive oil will produce an attractive and healthy gloss. The use of hot and cold water, alternating quickly from one application to the other, is of great value as a tonic for both hair and scalp, as it accelerates the circulation of the blood in the parts so treated.

Have the temperature of the heated water as hot as you can bear it, and the other as cold as possible without using ice; - hot and cold wet cloths applied alternately is a convenient substitute, if you cannot douse your head with the water itself. The change from hot to cold should be made at least five or six times at each treatment, but double that number will be beneficial and can do no harm. If life still remains in the roots of the hair a healthy growth will usually result. The tonic effect of this process is far more efficacious than any medicinal "hair invigorator" yet invented.

If the scalp is itchy, and there is a suspicion that microbes or germs of disease exist on it, dampen it with a carbolic acid wash. To one pint of water add a sufficient quantity of carbolic acid to produce, when the skin is moistened with the lotion, a very slight sensation of tingling, or heat. This treatment will, with daily applications, require about three weeks. It will surely destroy any germs of disease with which the scalp may be affected. It is an excellent tonic as well as an infallible and clean germicide, harmless, in the proportions advised, and superior to any advertised expensive their tonic or germicide which you may purchase.

When the hair is falling out many people are afraid to brush to wash it, fearing a still greater loss, and thinking to retain the dead hairs in the scalp. This is a serious mistake, as those dead hair roots, like any other decaying dead matter, are injurious to the healthy roots near them, and if allowed to remain increase the trouble. They should be removed for the same reason that decayed fruit is removed from its healthy neighbors. Dead and decaying mater is a menace to the life of a hair, just as, upon a larger scale, dead matter and unsanitary conditions are a menace to the life of a human being. In addition to these injurious effects of the dead roots, they impede the growth of new hairs which would spring up in the place of the dead ones, but which cannot do so while the dead roots remain. Remove the dead hairs as soon as possible, and other healthy hairs will replace them, springing from the same follicle, or root sheath.

The process is simple:

As I lie in bed I grasp my hair with my fingers, pulling gently, and changing the position of my hands until every part of the scalp has been treated. I alternate this pulling process by massaging the scalp with the tips of the fingers, which produces a perceptible glow, and has a general tonic effect, as it stimulates the circulation, and evidently determines the elements which feed the hair to the roots. By the hair-pulling process the scalp is lightly raised from the skull. The microscopic muscles and glands thus exercised, and obeying the general law of exercise, increase in size, strength, and elasticity, just as the larger muscles of the body are benefited by systematic exercise.

Go without your hat as much as possible. The practice is now popular, being a fashionable fad, and no longer specially noticeable. The sun has a very invigorating effect upon the hair. Baldness, among the races that do not wear hats, is almost unknown; but among the peasants or farmers in southern Germany, who wear their hats or caps day and night, baldness, without regard, without regard age, is the rule rather than the exception. I have lived in an Indian country and I do not remember of ever having seen a bald-headed Indian. That is a hint from nature.

Many people are afraid to use soap and water upon their hair, and quote self-constitute authorities in support of the statement that their use is injurious. Why should water be bad for the hair of the head but good for the hair of the beard or moustache! Such a contention is not logical, for the hair on the head and the hair on the face are identically the same; and it is certainly a most unusual occurrence for a man's beard to fall out unless caused by some local germ disease. That the beard is luxuriant in some individuals, while the scalp is devoid of hair, is to be accounted for by the fact that such men wash their faces and beard daily, and, in the drying process pull and exercise the roots; after which they brush it to keep it arranged. In this way they remove the dead hairs. As the skin is kept clean, by the face washing process, the conditions are favorable to the preservation of the hair upon that part of the head, even though the scalp may be bald.

Another mistaken belief is that when dandruff falls from the scalp it indicates a diseased condition. Dandruff is merely the exfoliation of the scarf, or outer skin, with the dried oil and waste matter thrown off by the glands.

The practice of the methods described will certainly relieve the trouble.

One of the arguments against washing the hair is that it causes or increases dandruff. The fact is, the dandruff was there before the scalp was washed, and the cleansing process merely dislodged it, so that its presence was more apparent.

Perspiration has a very injurious effect upon the hair. Athletes, especially, are sufferers from it, as they usually come in from long runs or other active exercise with the perspiration dripping from their every pore, the hair being as wet as the rest of the body. While particular efforts are made to bathe and cleanse every other part of their bodies, the scalp is neglected, the poisonous dead matter being allowed to remain and dry where it was eliminated. It is this neglect which is often noticeable among those whose excellent physical condition, due to athletic training, would seem to be a guarantee that the poor condition of their hair is not due to constitutional weakness.

Use daily is stiff brush; press the bristles well in; rub back and forth, and from side to side, thus loosening the dead skin, dried oil, etc., before trying to brush them off the head in the usual way.

Have the their trimmed often; the ends may split if this is neglected. Don't singe it. I do not believe the practice to be injurious, but it is simply a useless and expensive process, which can be better accomplished with the shears. The methods I have described are all logical; they are certainly inexpensive and easily performed, and I know from personal experience they are effective. Practice them as I have done and you need not fear the loss of your hair.

Deep-Breathing Exercise for the Development of the Lungs XLIII.

All of these exercises are perform in bed, under cover of the bed clothes

Deep-Breathing Exercises for the Development of the Lungs

A treatise upon the simple exercises and methods by which I am physically a young man at sixty-seven would be incomplete without a page upon breathing; for to breathe is to live, and "without breathe, there is no life". Differ as we may as to the virtues of the innumerable remedies and systems advocated throughout the world for the preservation of health, we all agree that life is absolutely dependent upon the act of breathing, and that man cannot be healthy unless this function is performed as nature intended.

At the commencement the infant draws a long, deep breath, instinctively retaining it to extract from the air its life-giving property; then exhales it in a long wail, and its life upon earth begins. At the end, with the chill of death upon him, the heart of the old man flutters faintly – then one gasp – he ceases to breathe, and the life principle, dependent upon that act, leaves the body forever. From the first faint breath of the infant, to the last gasp of the dying man, it is one long story of continued breathing, for life is but a series of breaths.

Man may exist for a month without eating, a much shorter time without drinking, but without breathing his existence upon the earth will be measured by a few – a very few – minutes. "Air is life," and without pure air good health is impossible; therefore keep in the open air as much as possible. See that your home is well ventilated, and sleep with your windows open. As you walk, frequently inhale deeply, feeling of dizziness, then exhale slowly, allowing the duration of inhalation and exhalation to be about equal. Practice this exercise as much as possible in the sunlight, for we are all dependent upon the sun for the life principle; its rays are filled with vibrations of energy and life, and the air vitalized by sunlight is an inexhaustible storehouse from which we extract the vital force as we breathe.

As you lie in bed in the morning, with the windows open, practice this deep-breathing exercise, the same movement as in walking. The most convenient position is upon your side or back.

It must be admitted that athletes or professional strong men are, as a rule, short lived, consumption and pneumonia being most frequently the cause of death among that class of men who, by reason of their strength and physical development, would seem to be immune from those diseases. Usually the sudden death of a noted athlete from pneumonia is attributed to dissipation after the arduous work of preparation for some athletic event, or undue exertion when "out of training". While this is often the case, it will not account for the deaths, by consumption and pneumonia, of a number of professional strong men, who were noted for their abstemious lives. The real reason has been that their bodies were unequally exercised; the external muscles being developed to their fullest capacity, but the lungs, being neglected, have remained in their original condition, and far inferior in their development to the powerful external structure. In this condition any unusual strain or exposure which might not have any deleterious effect upon the strong and thoroughly seasoned external muscles, might work very serious injury to the comparatively weak and poorly developed lungs. Like a chain, which is only as strong as its weakest link, this, the weakest part of the body, suffers.

If you would be healthy, developed the body evenly; and if these exercises for the lungs are practiced as described, you need not fear pulmonary diseases.

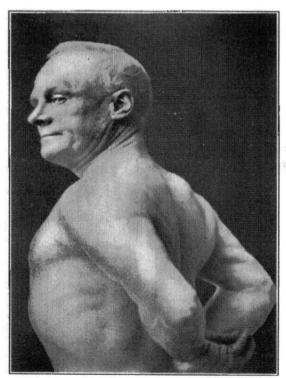

Chest Development, Showing Result of Deep-Breathing Exercise

I speak from experience, for my father died of consumption at the age of forty-two. I inherited weak lungs and a tendency to that dread disease. By these lung-strengthening exercises, I have increased the expansion of my chest from two and one-half inches of five and one-half inches, and am absolutely free from coughs, colds, or any lung weakness. I strongly urge the adoption of these deep-breathing exercises, or any other system of training or physical culture.

Cleanliness
External
XLIV.

**All of these exercises are perform in bed,
under cover of the bed clothes**

Cleanliness
External

The skin protects the soft and sensitive parts of the body from mechanical injury, and from the effects of heat or cold. It has over two million sweat tubes, aggregating several miles in length, through which it throws off from ten to fifteen thousand grains of dead matter daily. The under layer of skin is covered with a complete network of blood vessels spreading over a surface of nearly fifteen square feet.

There are also numerous oil glands which constantly throw off fatty secretions; an active, clean, healthy skin is, therefore, a very important factor in the process of eliminating dead and clogging matter, and in greatly aiding the work of the kidneys and lungs. It is essentially one of the principal conditions of health, while, on the other hand, an inert, dirty skin must necessarily increase the labor of the organs mentioned, hasten their decay, and shorten life. By profuse seating the weight of the body, when in a gross condition, and when there exists an excess of adipose tissue, can be reduce from two to five pounds in an hour.

When the skin is in an inert, stagnant condition, any sudden change in the atmosphere, which could have no injurious effect upon a healthy, vigorous skin, may produce a chill by which the secretions are checked, with the result that a large amount of blood may be driven to the interior and some of the organs may become congested. A bad cold, with all of its attendant discomforts, may follow, with the possibility even of other and more serious complications.

The necessity of keeping the pores open and free, to eliminate the waste matter, is quite evident, and the very best way to remove the surface dirt and accomplish the desired end is by the plentiful and frequent use of soap and warm water. Previous to the bath, create a friction on the back and shoulders and back of the legs with a rough Turkish towel, and on the chest, stomach, and front of the legs with horse-hair mittens, which can be purchased at almost any drug store. This will loosen the dead epidermic scales and the impurities lodged upon the skin, and greatly add to the benefit of the bath.

I advise the tepid bath; it is very true there is usually an invigorating effect in the cold bathwhere prompt reaction follows, but in the case of persons of advanced years, or those in poor health, recovery from the shock of cold water may not be prompt, and a distinct lowering of the vital force will temporarily follow. The face will appear drawn, and a sensation of exhaustion will be felt for some time afterwards; while, with the tepid bath, if the skin is previously subjected to vigorous friction – as described – the circulation will be accelerated, and the same tonic effect will be obtained, without any lowering of the nervous energy.

The water should be of about the same temperature as the skin.

If it be too hot, and the bath prolonged the muscles will relax and a feeling of lassitude will result. Therefore, my advice to those advanced in years, or in poor health, is to use the tepid bath as the "happy medium". Create a friction on the body as directed; then let there be a quick, but total, immersion. This practice daily will be sufficient to keep the skin in a healthy condition.

Cleanliness
Internal
XLV.

All of these exercises are perform in bed, under cover of the bed clothes

Cleanliness
Internal

I earnestly advise the "internal bath", - what is usually designated as "flushing the colon," or "rectal irrigation", - but most decidedly not what is known as taking an injection. Mere injections of a pint or a quart of water, as usually practiced, are insufficient and ineffective.

To properly wash the colon, at least four or five quarts of water are necessary, for the largest intestine is five feet in length, and when distended in fully three inches in diameter.

The proper appliance for cleaning the colon, or the large intestine, is a rubber water bag, with a capacity of five quarts, to which the injection pipe, or point, is attached at the center. The weight of the body forces the water into, and cleanses, the colon without the slightest physical effort. The time occupied in this operation is about fifteen minutes. It is the simplest and most effective appliance for this purpose yet invented, and is an important factor in my system of physical rejuvenation. I strongly advise its use at least once a weak. It is called "The Cascade", and is for sale by the Tyrrell Hygienic Institute, 1562 Broadway, New York. I cheerfully give the appliance this endorsement in return for the benefits I have derived from its use.

The importance of keeping this large intestine clear of obstruction is easily apparent. It is the receptacle for the waste matter of the system, and may be termed the sewer of the body. If it is allowed to become clogged with faecal matter, as is the case in constipation, it becomes the incubating ground of disease-breeding germs, and the source of all manner of diseases and complications, which would not occur if it were kept properly clean. Physic is but a poor method of attaining the end. The internal bath, by the process described, is the only logical, simple, and effective method by which it can be accomplished. To those who read this book and adopt my system of exercises. I strongly urge its practice, at least once a week, though twice a week is better.

Varicose Veins in the Legs – The Cause and the Cure XLVI.

All of these exercises are perform in bed, under cover of the bed clothes

Varicose Veins in the Legs – the Cause and the Cure

As we advance in years a distention of portions of the large veins in the legs in apt to appear. This is especially noticeable in the case of persons whose occupation necessitates a standing position, with little chance of exercise. Clerks, book-keepers, and workers at "the bench" in the different trades principally are the sufferers. This quiescent upright position produces stagnation of the blood in the legs; hence pressure and a steady strain upon the walls of the venous system at that point. Result, a permanent distention, or "varicose veins."

In youth, if a change of occupation is made, this affliction may disappear, but if the trouble ensues in or after middle age a cure by any lotion or other medicinal remedy is impossible.

It is true that a surgical operation will effect a cure, but that method of relief is expensive and painful, and will necessitate a discontinuance of occupation during the healing process. Temporary relief can be obtained by the use of an elastic stocking, but without this support a continuance of the occupation and position which caused the trouble will surely induce its return.

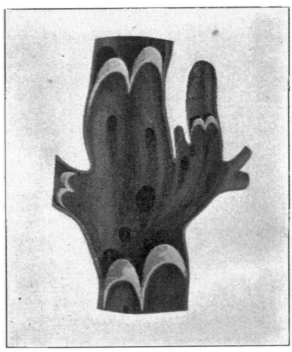

Valves of the Veins

The first indication of a varicose vein is a dull, aching pain. The vein becomes much larger, knotted, and distended; in extreme cases a rupture of the wall sometimes follows. This is infrequent, but always possible.

In the clinical report of my physical condition made by Doctor Carl Renz, February 5, 1895, which appears in the first pages of this book, he notes "various vein upon the inside of the right leg (uses an elastic stocking)". This affliction is a common one, is always annoying, and, writing from personal experience, often extremely painful.

It appeared when I had reached my fortieth year and annoyed me for eighteen years thereafter. I relieved myself of the trouble by the persistent practice of the simple exercise or method which I shall describe.

But first, to understand this method of cure, it is necessary to acquaint yourself with the structure of the weakened vein. You will then readily comprehend why the exercise. I practice and advise is beneficial. The following brief description of the venous system is a summary of a long chapter upon this subject taken from the standard text book – Gray's Anatomy. I have omitted the technical and scientific terms that the description may be readily understood by the average reader.

The veins are the vessels which serve to return the blood from the capillaries of the different parts of the body to the heart. The veins are found in nearly every tissue of the body. They are larger and altogether more numerous than the arteries; hence the entire capacity of the venous system is much greater than the arterials. The veins are not quite as cylindrical as the arteries, which are more dense in structure, stronger, more elastic, and preserve their cylindrical from when empty.

The veins have not this property, and collapse when not filled with blood. They have thinner walls than the arteries and are not so well supplied with muscular fibre; hence they are more liable to distention at any part where stagnation is liable to occur. All of the larger veins are provided valves. Their shape and position are shown in the accompanying illustration. These valves serve to prevent the reflux of the blood.

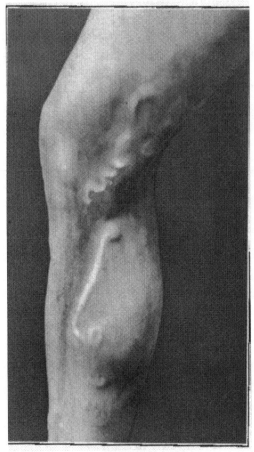

Varicose Veins

They are attached by their convex edges to the walls of the veins. Their concave margins are free and directed in the course of the venous current. They lie in close apposition with the wall of the vein as long as the current of blood takes its natural course. If, however, any stagnation or regurgitation occurs, the valves at that place become distorted, their opposed edges are brought into contact, the current is intercepted, and a distention of the wall of the vein ensues, which distention we know as that very painful affliction, a varicose vein.

As the primal cause of the trouble is stagnation of the blood at the point, acceleration of the circulation there would relieve that congestion; and the only way this can be effected is by friction. The most effective method of accomplishing this is with the dry palm of the hand, and the most convenient time and place is the same as in the other exercises I have described – in bed, and in the early morning. The conditions are then favorable, as the system is relaxed and will readily respond to intelligently directed efforts towards its rejuvenation or improvement.

The trouble will most probably appear upon the inside of the leg below the knee, running along the calf of the leg, but it may extend several inches above the knee and along the inside of the thigh. With increased years the congestion or distention of the superficial veins will extend lower down, immediately above and around the ankle. This may become discolored and assume a deep bluish hue because of the stagnant blood.

Relief is obtained by friction, with the palm of the hand, daily and persistently. This exercise will relieve the congestion, strengthen the minute muscles that support the venous walls, and if persisted in systematically and methodically, will finally restore the distorted venous valves to their proper position (see anatomical illustration facing page 114), when the trouble will disappear. It is a simple, easy, and effective remedy for a very annoying affliction. I speak from personal experience.

The most convenient position is lying upon your side. Commence with twenty strokes of the hand up and down, following the course of the vein, increasing as the skin becomes hardened and accustomed to the friction, to one hundred strokes. If persisted in, a cure is ultimately sure, in any ordinary case.

Rheumatism
XLVII.

All of these exercises are perform in bed, under cover of the bed clothes

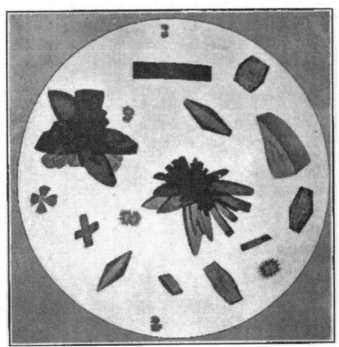

Uric Acid Crystals

Rheumatism

To those who have a tendency to acid rheumatism the methods I have described of eliminating the worn-out, or dead, matter from the system, are of great benefit. By this process of systematically exercising all the muscles of the body by alternate contractions and relaxations, the uric acid which is the basic cause of the trouble, and which the kidney have failed to eliminate, finds no place of permanent lodgment. It is compelled by the president agitation, to "move on," and is expelled by the natural excretions of the body before it has found time and place to settle and form into the minute crystals, which, like so many splinters, and are the cause of the acute pains characteristic of the diseases.

Rheumatism has been termed "the disease of age". This is not altogether true, for, while it must be admitted, that as we advance in years it is ever to be dreaded, to think that it is the inevitable disease of age is an error. It should be termed, rather, the disease of inaction and consequently disordered digestion.

The remedy is systematic muscular activity. In this way it is possible to eliminate from the system the cause of the disease. The simplest, most effective, and easiest method is described in these pages. I know from my own experience, and the experience of those who have followed my example, that this system of exercising every muscle of the body will surely prevent this most painful ailment; and, when it is not too far advanced, will effect a cure which may not be possible by the drug method.

In conclusion
XLVIII.

All of these exercises are perform in bed, under cover of the bed clothes

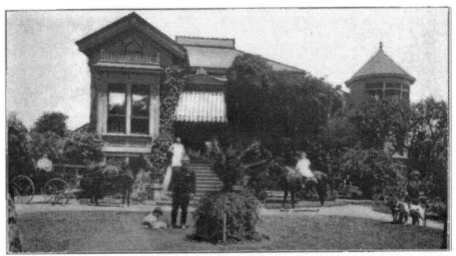

"Buens Vista", Home of Sanford Bennett, Alameds, California

In Conclusion

I have now described, as fully and clearly as I am capable of doing, the methods by which I have accomplished my physical rejuvenation, and why such a condition as mine, at sixty-seven, is possible by the system I practice. There is no question of my success, and I know the same satisfactory results are possible for anyone who will follow my example, - but will you do so! The majority will say, "that man has some good ideas", and add, "I feel that I do need a methodical system of exercise and when I have time I may take this up". You might as well say you have no time to eat or sleep. You can't be healthy unless you exercise. Health should be your first consideration. Financial success and other things are of secondary importance; for with health, strength, and elasticity of body the chances of financial success are greatly increased. Without these attributes, the greatest financial success is of but little value.

How many of our brain workers – our business men and professional men – have sacrificed health and happiness by following the paradox, "I am too busy – I haven't time to take care of my health"? There is only one result to a life upon these lines, - an early breakdown is inevitably certain. It is true that many have accomplished great wealth in exchange for their health, but have spent that wealth in vainly endeavoring to regain their former, but now wasted, physical vigor.

I don't decry financial success. Wealth is a very good thing to have; but the greatest financial success will not compensate for ill health. Better stop now, before it is too late, and take the time to make yourself strong; for otherwise you may be forced to attend your own funeral, brought about prematurely by lack of muscular activity and other violations of the laws of Nature.

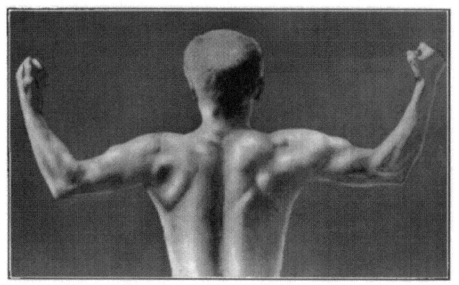

Sanford Bennett at 56

Another objection often raised is, "I am too old". To this I have already made my answer. If I, a chronic dyspeptic at fifty, with adverse hereditary and physical conditions and unfavorable environments, have been able, by the simple methods I have described, to build myself up and to acquire the strength, elasticity of body, and vital energy I now possess, but never had in the best days of my youth, then you, too, can surely have the same success. You are not too old. Try it. Commence now, and you will succeed.

"Too much trouble" – that is the objection of a lazy person. If, by the same exertions for one year, you could be assured that you would receive $50,000, you would not think that too much trouble, but would esteem it the opportunity of your life. Yet the health, and improved physical condition, which would surely result from one year's systematic and persistent practice of the methods I have described, could not be purchased for that or any other sum.

It is true that to be in the best physical condition does require unremitting attention; but the end is worth the means, for the reward is health, strength, elasticity of body, and longevity, - the real, the greatest, riches in the world. Just as engineers and expert machinist, employed to care for the intricate machinery of a great ocean steamship, are forever polishing up and looking after the various details of that machinery, that they may have its highest efficiency; so the complicated machinery of the human body must be assiduously and intelligently cared for, or it will surely deteriorate.

There is not "royal road to health". It cannot be bought; if you would possess it, you must work for it.

But the way is easy, the work not hard. As you lie comfortably in bed tomorrow morning, commence the practice of any one of the muscular contractions and relaxations I have described, and, when you have learned that, take up the next. Finally you will have acquired and entire system, which you will find to be an easy, certain, and inexpensive method of acquiring health.

An illustrated chart accompanies this book. Hang it near your bed, where you can easily see the positions described in the exercises. You will find them easily learned. Commence tomorrow morning.

There is a very popular form of printed advice which you frequently find hanging over desks in business houses: "Do IT Now".

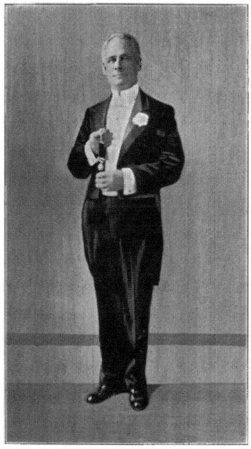

"I move We Adjourn"

For more old time classics of strength, visit:

STRONGMANBOOKS.COM

*Sign up on the website for a free gift and
updates about new books added regularly.*

Titles Available About and From All These Authors:

Arthur Saxon	William Blaikie
Bob Hoffman	Farmer Burns
Maxick	Monte Saldo
Eugen Sandow	Lionel Strongfort
George F. Jowett	Antone Matysek
Otto Arco	Harry Paschall
George Hackenschmidt	Louis Cyr
Thomas Inch	Alois Swoboda
Edward Aston	William Pullum
Bernarr MacFadden	Joe Bonomo
Earle Liederman	Siegmund Breitbart
Alan Calvert	Mighty Apollon
Alexander Zass	And Many More

Made in the USA
Columbia, SC
29 February 2024

32483236R00070